Evaluation of Potential Employee Exposures During Crime and Death Investigations at a County Coroner's Office

Bradley S. King, MPH, CIH;
Kristin Musolin, DO, MS;
JungHo Choi, MS

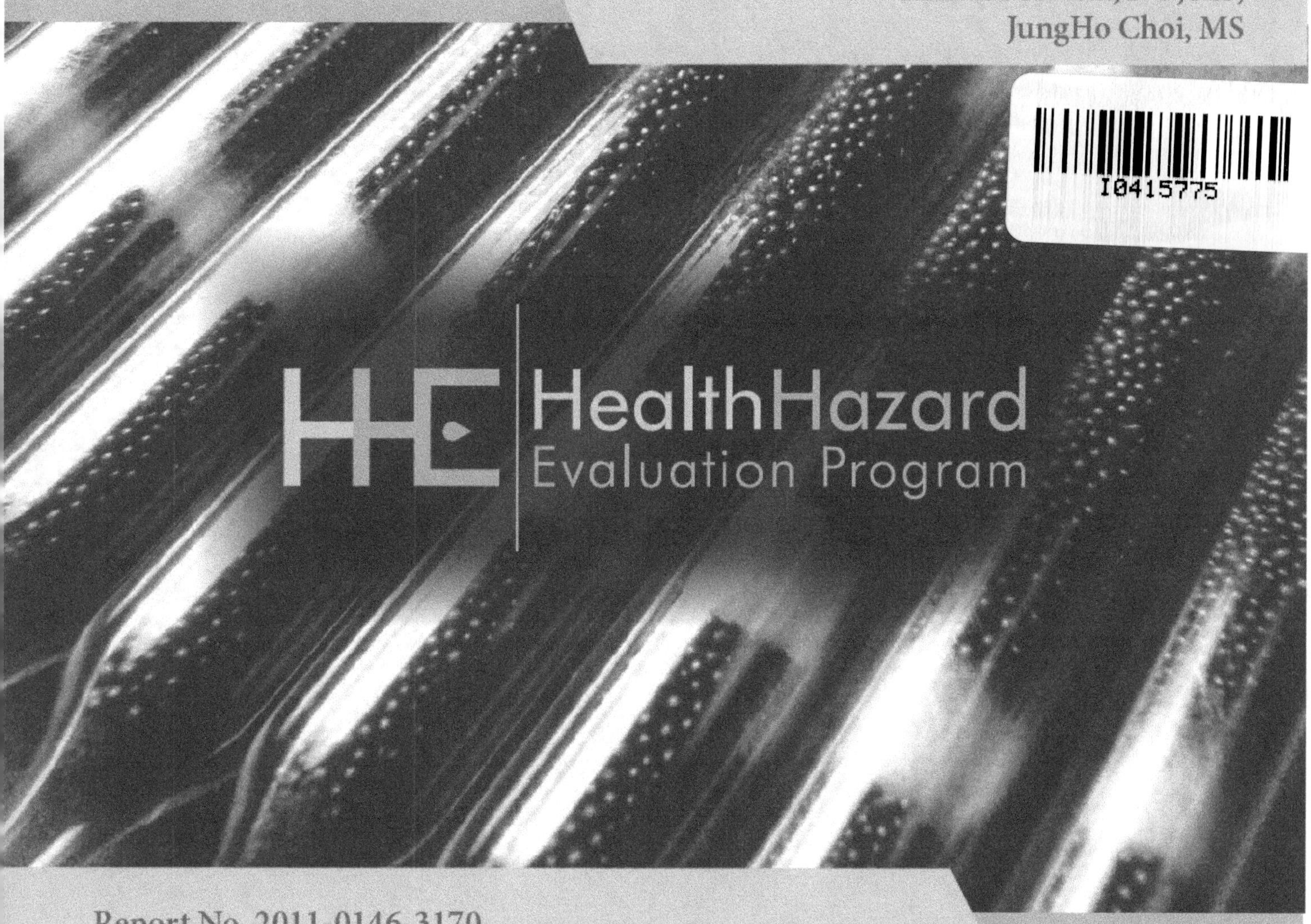

HealthHazard Evaluation Program

I0415775

Report No. 2011-0146-3170
March 2013

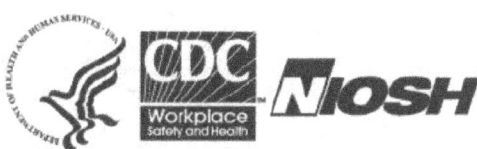

U.S. Department of Health and Human Services
Centers for Disease Control and Prevention
National Institute for Occupational Safety and Health

CDC Workplace Safety and Health

NIOSH

Contents

Highlights of this Evaluation

The Health Hazard Evaluation Program received a request from a coroner's office in Ohio. The employer wanted to determine if conditions and work practices at the facility were posing a health hazard to employees.

What We Did

- We evaluated the facility in October 2011. We returned in January 2012 to complete our evaluation.

- We interviewed employees about their work and health. These interviews were confidential.

- We observed work practices and procedures in the autopsy suite, histology laboratory, fingerprint evidence laboratory, drug evidence laboratory, and firearms section.

- We sampled the air for formaldehyde and airborne particles during six autopsy procedures.

- We sampled the air for formaldehyde and volatile organic compounds. These samples were taken in the histology laboratory during tissue prepping and processing.

- We took air samples for ethyl 2-cyanoacrylate. These samples were taken during fingerprint fuming operations.

- We took samples for residual drug particles. These samples were collected from the air and work surfaces in the drug evidence laboratory.

- We sampled for lead. These samples were collected from the air and work surfaces in the firearms section.

- We evaluated the ventilation system in several areas.

> We evaluated potential exposures among investigators at a county coroner's office. We found that some exposures to formaldehyde in the autopsy suite exceeded recommended exposure levels. Lead contamination of surfaces in the firearms section and drug particle contamination of surfaces in the drug evidence laboratory may pose a health hazard. Recommendations are provided to improve work conditions and minimize exposures.

What We Found

- Employees reported few health symptoms that they thought were related to their work.

- Some exposures to formaldehyde in the autopsy suite were above recommended ceiling limits.

- The number of air changes per hour in the autopsy suite was below recommended levels.

- Exposures to formaldehyde in the histology laboratory were below recommended ceiling limits. Air sampling for volatile organic compounds in the histology laboratory showed low levels of organic compounds commonly found in the indoor environment.

- Exposures to ethyl 2-cyanoacrylate during latent fingerprint development were low.

What We Found (continued)

- Airborne drug particles were found in the samples taken during drug analyses. Drug particles were also found on surfaces in the drug evidence laboratory.

- Air did not flow from the shooter towards the target in the firing room as recommended for firing ranges.

- Airborne concentrations of lead may be a health hazard to firearm examiners if they do multiple sessions of weapon testing during a work shift.

- We found lead contamination on surfaces in the firing room. The presence of lead could be a potential health hazard.

What the Employer Can Do

- Increase room exhaust in the autopsy suite. This will increase the number of air changes per hour in that area.

- Install downdraft tables in the autopsy suite to help control formaldehyde exposures.

- Modify the supply and exhaust ventilation in the firing room to provide a laminar flow of air that passes from the shooter towards the bullet trap. Until modifications are made, limit the number of weapons tested in any one day.

- Perform procedures that could produce airborne particles of drugs under a high-efficiency particulate air filtered hood.

- Clean contaminated surfaces in the drug evidence laboratory and firearm examiners' firing room.

- Improve housekeeping practices to prevent build-up of surface contamination of lead in the firing room. This is also true for preventing build-up of drug particles in the drug evidence laboratory.

- Use high-efficiency particulate air filtered vacuum or wet mopping methods to clean the firing range. Do not dry sweep in the firing range.

- Ensure exhaust vents are not blocked in the autopsy suites.

- Sample for lead and formaldehyde. This should be done as a follow-up to see if levels have changed after work practices are changed or controls introduced.

- Provide employees with recommended personal protective equipment including respirators, lab coats, gloves, safety goggles or glasses, and face shields. Make sure that employees are using this equipment for specific work practices taking place in the facility.

What Employees Can Do

- Use local exhaust ventilation attachments when using the saw for cranial autopsies.

- Only open containers of formaldehyde when needed during autopsies.

What Employees Can Do (continued)

- Wash your hands with warm water and soap after completing work activities. Always wash after autopsies, weapon testing, and drug analysis.

- Report any symptoms that you think may be related to your work to a supervisor. If you have concerns about safety, report those also.

- Become active in the health and safety committee. Attend meetings and take any training that is related to your job.

- Wear personal protective equipment that is recommended for the task you are doing.

- Wear an N95 respirator approved by the National Institute for Occupational Safety and Health during autopsies.

Abbreviations

µg	Micrograms
µg/cm^2	Micrograms per square centimeter
µg/dL	Micrograms per deciliter
µg/m^3	Micrograms per cubic meter
µm	Micrometer
ACGIH®	American Conference of Governmental Industrial Hygienists
BLL	Blood lead level
C	Ceiling limit
CDC	Centers for Disease Control and Prevention
cfm	Cubic feet per minute
CFR	Code of Federal Regulations
HHE	Health hazard evaluation
NAICS	North American Industry Classification System
ND	Not detected
ng/cm^2	Nanograms per square centimeter
ng/m^3	Nanograms per cubic meter
NIOSH	National Institute for Occupational Safety and Health
OEL	Occupational exposure limit
OSHA	Occupational Safety and Health Administration
PEL	Permissible exposure limit
ppm	Parts per million
REL	Recommended exposure limit
TLV®	Threshold limit value
TWA	Time-weighted average
WEEL™	Workplace environmental exposure level

Introduction

The National Institute for Occupational Safety and Health (NIOSH) received a health hazard evaluation (HHE) request from managers at a county coroner's office in Ohio. The request concerned possible health hazards associated with work practices in several sections including the autopsy suite of the coroner's office during post-mortem examinations and various sections of the crime laboratory during the analysis of evidence related to criminal investigations. We evaluated the facility on October 7, 2011; October 20, 2011; and January 10–12, 2012.

Facility Description

The coroner's office occupied a four-story building completed in 1973. At the time of the evaluation, the office employed approximately 50 full-time and part-time staff. Two autopsy suites, coolers, a morgue, storage, and office areas occupied the first floor of the building. Administrative offices were on the second floor. The third floor housed the following sections of the crime laboratory: histology, toxicology, serology, firearms, trace evidence, arson, and documents. The fourth floor housed mechanical equipment. Separate air handling systems serviced the first three floors. On the first floor, the air handling system was a constant volume system designed to supply 10,800 cubic feet per minute (cfm) of air, providing eight different temperature control zones. Air supplied to the autopsy suites was exhausted directly outdoors, while air supplied to the first floor storage and offices areas was returned to the air handling unit for recirculation. The air handling system for the second floor was a constant volume system with a dual duct design to distribute 13,200 cfm of hot and cold conditioned air to terminal boxes where they were mixed to provide for temperature control for that area of the floor. Air was returned to the air handling unit from most spaces on this floor. For the third floor, the air handling system was a constant volume system also designed as a dual duct system that supplied 12,600 cfm of air. In general, air supplied to the laboratories was exhausted directly outside the building while air supplied to corridors and office areas was recirculated. However, because of space needs, laboratory functions were performed in some areas originally designed and used for office functions.

Work Process Descriptions

Employees in the coroner's office performed a wide variety of specialized work processes to provide forensic services that supported local police investigations.

In the autopsy suite, official autopsies were conducted for deaths from homicide, suicide, fires/ burns, certain accidents, and other suspicious or unusual deaths. During a typical autopsy, a pathologist and forensic assistant opened the decedent's chest cavity to remove and examine the internal organs. Organ tissue samples were removed and placed in open containers of a formalin solution containing 37% formaldehyde in water and methanol. This solution was used to fix and preserve the tissue specimens for histologic examination. To gain access to the brain tissue, the skull cap of the decedent was removed with a hand-held oscillating Clean Cut Autopsy Saw system, model 04-NS3 (Leica Microsystems, Buffalo Grove, Illinois [formerly

Surgipath Medical Industries, Richmond, Illinois]). No local exhaust ventilation system was employed when the bone-cutting oscillating saw was used.

Tissues collected during autopsies were fixed, processed, embedded in paraffin wax, sectioned, mounted on a slide, and stained for microscopic examination of the tissue cells in the histology laboratory. Following autopsies, these tissues were delivered to the laboratory in containers of 100–300 milliliters of formalin solution containing 37% formaldehyde. The tissues, contained in small cassettes, were removed from the containers and loaded into a tray for further processing. Typically, this work was done near a hood on the wall directly above the sink into which the formalin waste was poured after the cassettes were removed (Figure 1). Processing of the tissues sequentially removed the tissue fluids and replaced them with alcohol and paraffin so that the tissue was fixed in a block of paraffin. Chemicals used in the tissue processing included dehydrants such as ethyl, isopropyl, and methyl alcohol, and aliphatic hydrocarbons. The total time for loading tissue cassettes and tissue processing was 1–1.5 hours; this occurred once every other week at a minimum to twice a week at a maximum. After processing, the block was sliced, and the tissue specimens were mounted on a slide, stained, and viewed under a microscope.

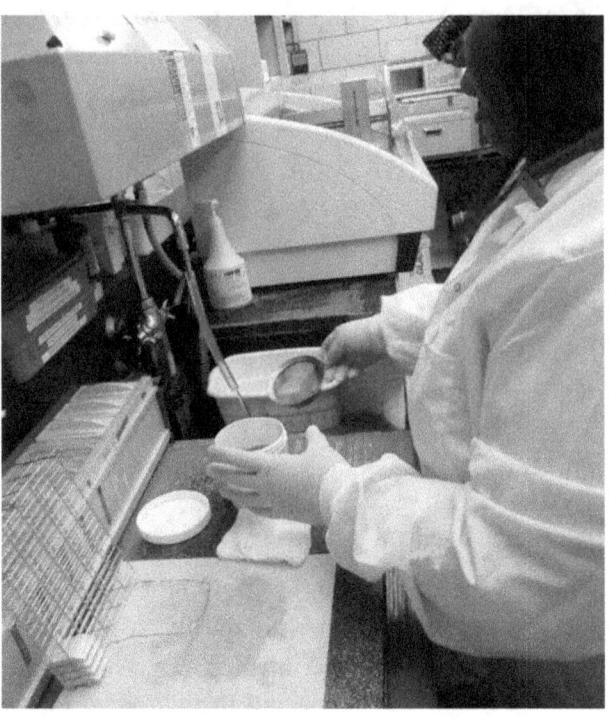

Figure 1. A histologist prepares to drain the formalin from a container through a strainer. The strainer catches the tissue cassettes prior to their placement in the processing tray.

In the fingerprint evidence laboratory, a latent fingerprint development process was used to recover fingerprints on a variety of evidentiary materials and objects. Several methods were available including the use of cyanoacrylate adhesive glue (super glue) fuming. The super glue used in this method contained more than 50% ethyl 2-cyanoacrylate. In this process, the object with the fingerprint on it was hung in a fuming chamber (Figure 2). A small

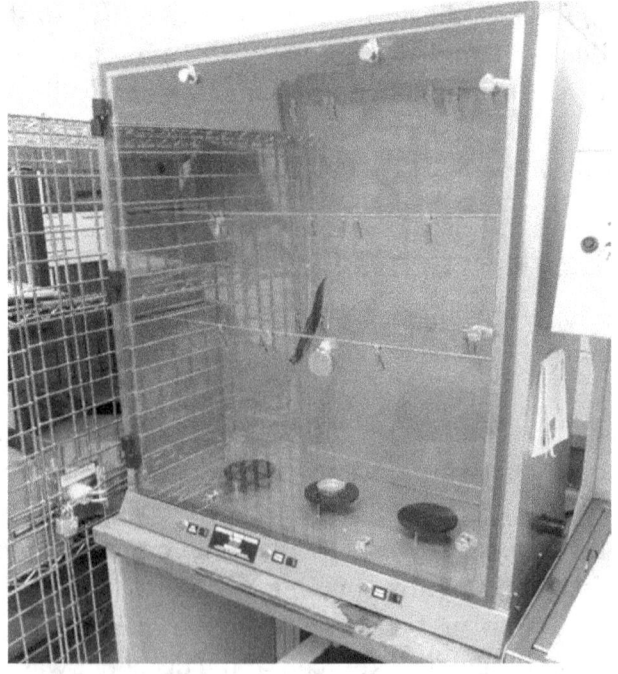

Figure 2. A super glue fuming chamber for fingerprint development with a suspended knife inside.

quantity of super glue was placed in a shallow open container at the bottom of the chamber. After the chamber door was closed, the super glue was heated to create gaseous cyanoacrylate that adhered to the fingerprint secretions on the object. Once the object was removed from the chamber after the process was complete, the fixed fingerprint was dyed with a fluorescent substance, examined under ultraviolet light, and photographed. The fingerprint specialist reported that latent fingerprint development tasks were performed 1–2 times per week on average, with 1–2 items per run.

Chemical identification and confirmation of confiscated drugs were done in the drug evidence laboratory. Samples were analyzed by drug analysts to determine the type and amount of drugs (Figure 3). Examples of drugs analyzed by the laboratory include marijuana, cocaine, heroin, methamphetamine, and pharmaceutical opioids (e.g., oxycodone, methadone). Drugs may have been present in several forms including powders, pills, and plant material; as injectable liquids; or as residues on objects such as syringes and pipes. Much of the analytical work was performed on a laboratory bench top. Four chemical fume hoods with ducted exhaust to the outside were in the laboratory as well as a ductless high-efficiency particulate air filtered hood that was used to open large (i.e., typically larger than 1 kilogram) packages of drugs.

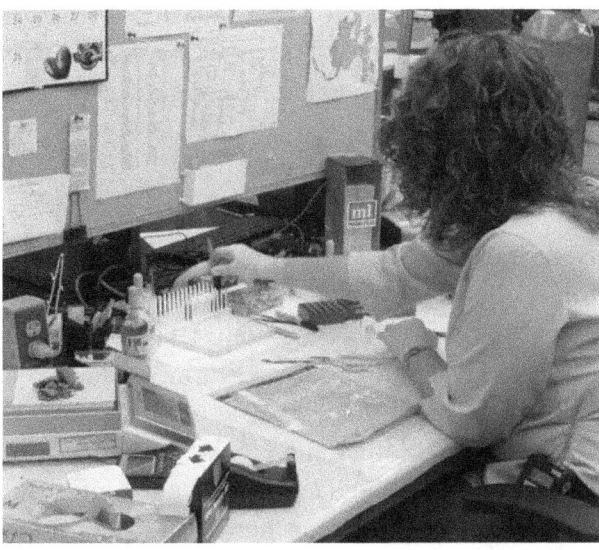

Figure 3. A drug analyst analyzes a sample of illicit drugs.

Examinations of firearms and ammunition used in crimes were done in the firearms section. Within the firearms section, weapons were fired in two locations: a narrow work room with a bullet trap at one end (Figure 4) and a water tank in a garage on the first floor (Figure 5). The water tank was used when the analyst needed to retrieve bullets for analysis. The bullet trap in the firing room was last cleaned in April 2010. For a typical case investigation, two shots per gun were required, with each case taking approximately 2 hours. Up to four cases may be investigated on a busy day, requiring the firing of weapons 10–12 times in a day.

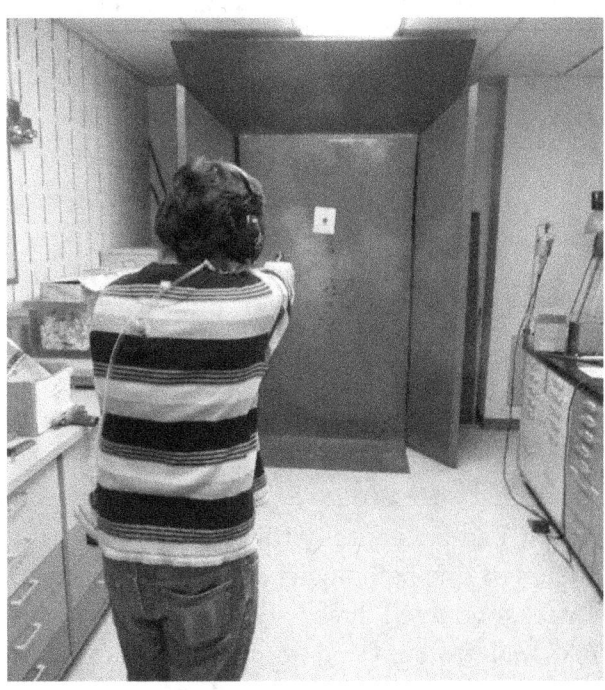

Figure 4. The firearms examiner fires a weapon into the bullet trap. The photo shows the visible cloud of airborne particles produced when firing.

In addition to work described above, specialized work in other areas included serology investigations of dried biological fluid and deoxyribonucleic acid testing; toxicology investigations of drugs and poisons in body fluids and tissues; evaluation of trace evidence such as the analysis or comparison of hairs, fibers, particles, or residues; and analysis of evidence related to arson investigations.

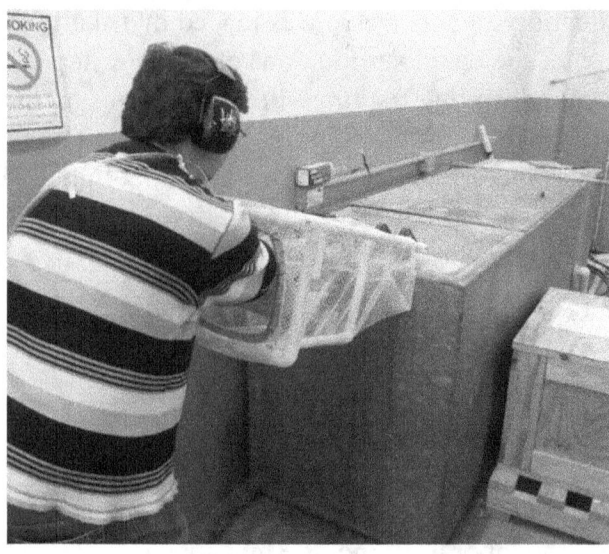

Figure 5. The firearms examiner fires a weapon into the water tank.

Methods

Before our initial site visit, we reviewed the following documents: a list of current employees, copies of the Ohio Bureau of Workers' Compensation Form 300P Logs of Work-Related Injuries and Illnesses from 2006–2010, the safety manual, a list of Occupational Safety and Health Administration (OSHA) training videos, and employee blood lead level (BLL) and audiometric testing results from 2005, 2007, and 2010. On October 7, 2011, we visited the coroner's office and met with employer and employee representatives to discuss the concerns described in the request. We toured the first floor autopsy suites and the third floor laboratory sections. During the tour, we observed work processes, practices, and workplace conditions and spoke briefly with employees in each area. We discussed and reviewed the facility's safety plan and training programs as well as material safety data sheets for a variety of chemicals. On October 20, 2011, we returned to hold confidential medical interviews with 14 of 49 employees regarding health and workplace concerns.

On the basis of our observations and review of the information provided, we returned to the facility to conduct exposure assessments on January 10–12, 2012, in the autopsy suite, the histology laboratory, the fingerprint evidence laboratory, the drug evidence laboratory, and the firearms section. Details of the methods used during the exposure assessments are included in Appendix A of this report. Diagrams of areas evaluated, including airflow measurements and locations of surface wipe samples, are included in Appendix B.

Autopsy Suite

On January 10, 2012, we observed six autopsies in autopsy suite 1 on the first floor. Autopsy suite 1 had the capacity for two simultaneous autopsies, with each autopsy performed by a team of one pathologist and one forensic assistant. On the day of the evaluation, two teams conducted three back-to-back autopsies each. We observed the teams' work practices. Personal protective equipment worn during autopsies included N95 filtering face piece respirators, surgical masks, safety glasses, face shields, latex gloves, aprons with sleeves, scrubs, booties, and head covers. Personal breathing zone air samples were taken for formaldehyde on the two pathologists and on the two forensic assistants. One pathologist wore the same sampling equipment over the course of the three autopsies to collect a longer-term sample; the sampling equipment on the other pathologist was changed at the end of each autopsy to collect shorter-term, tasked-based samples. Task-based samples during each autopsy were taken on both of the forensic assistants. A general area air sample was collected on one of the autopsy tables over the time that work was going on in the autopsy suite. Because the oscillating saw used during the autopsies can create considerable quantities of airborne particulate matter, a direct-reading real-time aerosol monitor (Met One HHPC-6 Handheld Airborne Particle Counter [Hach Ultra Analytics, Grants Pass, Oregon]) was placed above one of the autopsy tables to measure the concentration of airborne particles. We used an AccuBalance Plus model 8373 air capture hood (TSI Inc., Shoreview, Minnesota) after the autopsies were completed to determine the number of air changes per hour in the autopsy suite, and we used smoke tubes (Nextteq, Tampa, Florida) to visualize air flow patterns.

Histology Laboratory

On January 11, 2012, we assessed exposures in the histology laboratory where human tissue specimens collected during autopsies were received and processed. We observed the histologist's work practices while she prepared, processed, and fixed tissues delivered from previous autopsies. Personal protective equipment worn during these tasks included powder-free latex gloves and a laboratory coat. She also wore non-safety prescription glasses. A task-based breathing zone sample for formaldehyde was collected on the histologist while she changed chemicals in the tissue processor, removed tissue cassettes from the formalin-holding containers, and placed the cassettes in the processing tray. These activities took about 1–1.5 hours. General area air samples were also taken during these tasks for formaldehyde and volatile organic compounds in areas around the histology laboratory. The histologist did not load or process tissues for the rest of the day outside of this sampling period.

Fingerprint Evidence Laboratory

On January 11, 2012, we observed the latent fingerprint specialist as he developed a latent fingerprint on a knife. Personal protective equipment worn during this task included nitrile gloves and a laboratory coat. A task-based breathing zone air sample was taken on the specialist for ethyl 2-cyanoacrylate during this activity. General area air samples for ethyl 2-cyanoacrylate were collected inside and outside the room during the hour that he worked. The fingerprint specialist did not develop fingerprints for the rest of the day outside of this sampling period.

Drug Evidence Laboratory

On January 12, 2012, we assessed exposures in the drug evidence laboratory that received samples of illicit drugs and drug paraphernalia collected at crime scenes. We observed work practices of three drug analysts working at their bench top work locations. They wore nitrile gloves during these activities; one analyst wore non-safety prescription glasses. Each analyst evaluated 10–12 cases on the day of the monitoring. Because a case may involve multiple samples, the total number of drug samples analyzed per analyst on this day was 21–36. Task-based breathing zone air samples were taken for airborne drug particles on each of the three analysts during this work. Two general area air samples in the drug evidence laboratory were taken during these activities, as was one area air sample in the drug storage vault. The analysts did not analyze drugs for the rest of the day outside of this sampling period. Several wipe samples for drug particles were taken from work surfaces throughout the drug evidence laboratory to investigate potential contamination with drug residues.

Firearms Section

On January 12, 2012, we observed work practices in the firearms section. During the 60-minute sampling period on the day of our assessment, the firearms examiner twice fired a .45 caliber automatic pistol with 230-grain copper full metal jacket bullets and twice fired a .38 caliber revolver with 158-grain lead rounds. These were shot directly into the bullet trap in the firearms room. Additionally, the firearms examiner shot the .45 caliber pistol once into the water tank. Personal protective equipment worn during these activities included safety glasses, ear muffs, and ear plugs; employees could select to wear one or both of the hearing protection devices. Lab coat use was discretionary. A task-based breathing zone air sample was taken on the firearms examiner for airborne lead during the period when he fired these weapons. General area air samples for lead were also collected inside and outside the weapons firing room while he conducted weapons firing. The firearms examiner did not fire weapons for the rest of the day outside of this sampling period. Nine wipe samples for lead were taken on the floor and work surfaces inside and outside the weapons firing room, at the water tank, and on the hands of the firearms examiner after he completed the series of weapon firings. Using the same methods we used in the autopsy suite, we measured the amount of air supplied to and exhausted from the firearms room and determined directional air flow patterns within the room and between the firearms room and an adjacent room.

Results

Employee Interviews and Record Review

On October 20, 2011, we held voluntary, confidential medical interviews with a convenience sample of 14 of 49 employees. Interviewees included 9 women and 5 men; ages ranged from 24–64 years, with an average of 41 years. We asked a series of questions about their job description, work practices, personal protective equipment use, and work-related health and safety concerns.

Interviewed employees worked in the clerical office; the autopsy suite; and the histology, drug evidence, fingerprint evidence, trace evidence, firearms, toxicology, and serology laboratories. Some interviewed employees also worked off-site at death scene investigation locations. Although medico-legal death investigators were interviewed, we did not evaluate death scene investigation locations for logistical reasons. Most employees worked approximately 40 hours a week, 9.5 hours a day, taking one day off every other week. The forensic medical assistants worked a rotating schedule of varying lengths of days on and off in order to have a minimum of three employees on duty at a time. The number of years worked at the facility ranged from 1 to 24 years, with an average of 10 years.

Of the 14 employees we interviewed, 10 reported concerns they felt were related to the workplace. These included general building ventilation concerns and lack of exhaust for the latent fingerprint chamber, overcrowding, stress related to budget cuts, and exposure to potentially harmful chemicals. Eight employees reported a history of seasonal allergies. Self-reported symptoms that employees felt were related to work included headaches in two employees, and work-related stress in one employee. Self-reports of work-related injuries included needlestick injuries (four employees), cuts from a scalpel blade (two employees), and eye splash (one employee). According to the employees, the needlestick injuries were reported and followed-up medically. Two employees were exposed to blood borne pathogens through contaminated needles (Hagedorn needles used for suturing, and intravenous needles used for drawing blood), two through contaminated scalpel and microtome blades, and one as a result of a water splash from the autopsy table. Gloves were worn during all incidents, but face shield use was initiated after the eye splash injury.

The Logs for 2006–2010 included four injuries and two illnesses. Cuts were the most common event, accounting for 50% of reports. Fingers were the most commonly affected body part; other injuries and illnesses included contusions and a foreign body in the eye.

The employer provided personal protective equipment for employees. Employees reported wearing either latex or nitrile gloves for the following duties: opening evidence and drug packages, handling and mixing chemicals, handling serology material and biohazards, conducting death scene investigations, and removing personal items from bodies. Employees also said they used surgical masks when opening bags with large quantities of illicit drugs. The firearms examiners reported wearing either earmuffs only or both earmuffs and ear plugs when test firing weapons. All employees working in the autopsy suite reported that they wore either safety goggles or a face shield. Current policy at the facility was the voluntary use of respirators during activities such as autopsies. Employees specifically reported wearing NIOSH-approved N95 filtering facepiece respirators during autopsies of individuals suspected of having had tuberculosis.

Each autopsy employee who operated the x-ray machine wore a dosimeter that monitored for radiation exposure and was read by an outside company every 3 months. Firearms examiners received a blood lead analysis and an audiogram to test hearing every 5 years. We evaluated the most recent results of BLL and zinc protoporphyrin for the three employees who worked in the firearms section. The three tests we reviewed showed BLLs below 2.6 micrograms per deciliter (µg/dL) and zinc protoporphyrin levels below 29 µg/dL, with no evidence of excessive body absorption of lead from 2007–2010. Lead testing appeared to be in compliance with the OSHA lead standard in regards to baseline and continued testing of BLL and zinc protoporphyrin. We evaluated audiograms from all firearms examiners from 2010 (two employees) and from 2007 (one employee) and found no evidence of noise-induced hearing loss. However, one employee reported during the interview that he/she did not receive the BLL and audiometric testing results.

Autopsy Suite

We collected task-based personal breathing zone and area air samples for formaldehyde during six autopsies in autopsy suite 1 (Table 1). Sampling times ranged from 54 to 238 minutes. All short-term personal breathing zone air sample results for formaldehyde were at or above the NIOSH ceiling limit of 0.1 parts per million (ppm) [NIOSH 2010b]. One of the forensic assistant's breathing zone air sample results exceeded the American Conference of Governmental Industrial Hygienists (ACGIH®) ceiling limit of 0.3 ppm [ACGIH 2012].

Table 1. Air sampling results for formaldehyde collected in autopsy suite 1 on January 10, 2012

Sample location	Sample type	Sampling period (minutes)	Concentration (ppm)
Pathologist 1	PBZ	67	0.28
	PBZ	Equipment failure	Not applicable
	PBZ	54	0.13
Pathologist 2	PBZ	233	0.27
Forensic assistant 1	PBZ	102	0.29
	PBZ	54	0.15
	PBZ	83	0.10
Forensic assistant 2	PBZ	98	0.46
	PBZ	80	0.23
	PBZ	72	0.15
Autopsy table	GA	238	0.18
NIOSH REL			C 0.1
ACGIH TLV			C 0.3

PBZ = personal breathing zone
GA = general area
C = ceiling

Real-time aerosol measurements were taken with direct-reading instrumentation mounted above one of the autopsy tables (Figure B1). As shown in Figure 6, background aerosol concentrations (measured in particles per liter of air) begin at 8:43 a.m., before any autopsy procedures began. Most particles measured were 0.3–0.5 micrometers (µm) in diameter. The major source of additional aerosols produced during the autopsies was the use of the oscillating saw to cut through the cranial bone to remove the skull cap. No local exhaust ventilation was used during this procedure. Aerosol concentrations peaked when the saw was used during each autopsy. Typically, bone cutting with the saw lasted no longer than 5 minutes. Figure 6 shows three solid-line boxes that represent the time when the oscillating saw was used at the autopsy table where the particle counter was mounted. Figure 6 also shows three dashed-line boxes that represent the time when

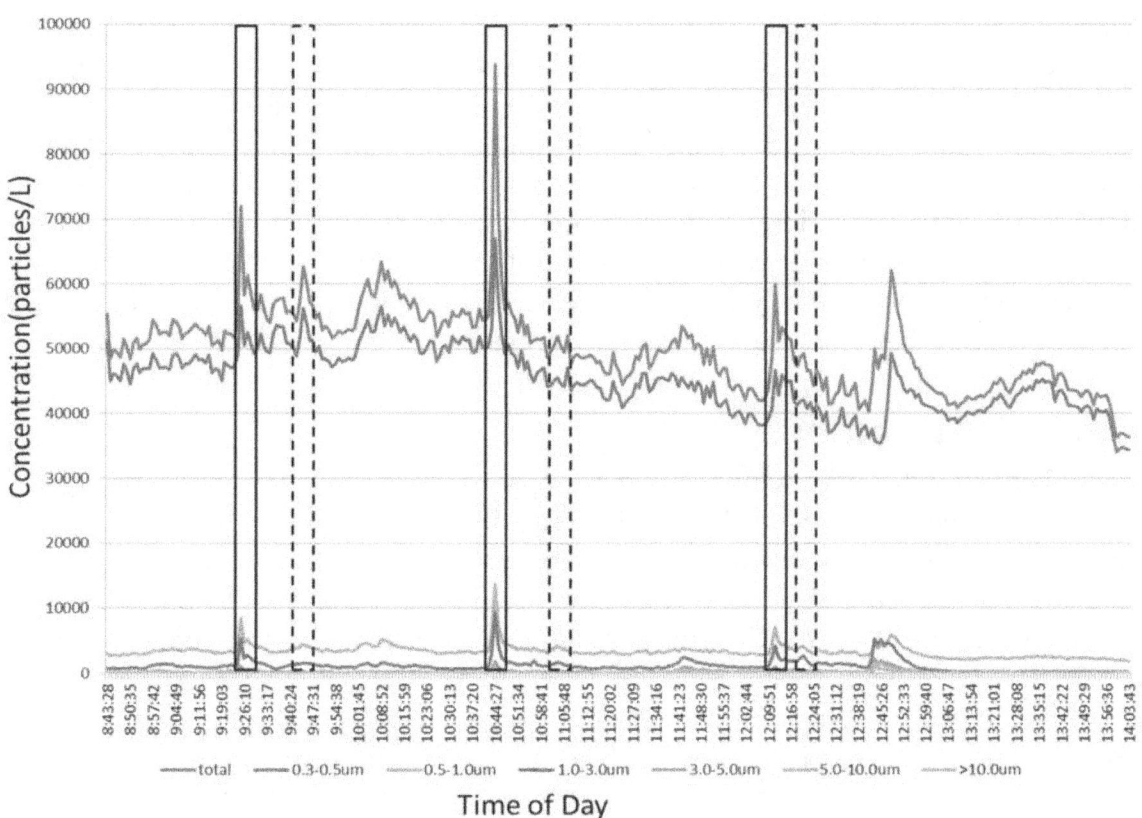

Figure 6. Concentration of aerosols in autopsy suite during six autopsies.

the oscillating saw was used at the second autopsy table on the opposite side of the autopsy suite. Although peaks were observed while the saws were in use, aerosol levels returned to background levels fairly rapidly after the saws were turned off. A peak observed between 12:45 p.m. and 12:50 p.m. corresponded with activities related to completion of the day's autopsy activities such as the final cleaning of the suite.

Ventilation measurements were taken at each of the supply and exhaust vents within the autopsy suite (Figure B1). The two supply vents were in the autopsy suite ceiling directly above the autopsy tables. Together they supplied 521 cfm of air to the room. Two vents in opposite corners of the suite exhausted air from the room directly outside. Combined, these two vents exhausted 431 cfm of air. We observed exhaust vents in the autopsy room blocked by boxes, trash bins, and other equipment that likely reduced their effectiveness. On the basis of the exhaust measurements and the measured dimensions of the autopsy suite, the calculated number of air changes per hour for the room was 5.4.

Observations made during autopsies revealed work practices that may increase the risk of sharps injuries. We observed some employees holding skin flaps with her hands instead of using forceps while suturing with string to close the skull cap and the chest cavity at the end of an autopsy. When filling test tubes with blood, vitreous fluid, or urine collected with a syringe, we observed a worker holding the test tube directly with their hands, increasing the chances of a needlestick injury when inserting the syringe into the tube. Autopsy personnel were observed to use their hands to put on and take off the blades of reusable scalpels instead of using forceps or a hemostat. Furthermore, neither disposable safety scalpels nor automatic blade removal devices for reusable scalpels were used. This was in contrast to our observations in the histology laboratory where the histologist used a scalpel blade removal device that automatically removed and sealed used blades inside a puncture-resistant container without the need to remove the blade from the scalpel by hand. We also observed that the sharps container in the autopsy suite was almost completely filled. Some autopsy employees chose to wear a surgical mask instead of an N95 filtering facepiece respirator; respirators were used voluntarily. Additionally, we observed that at least one employee did not wear booties to cover their shoes while in the autopsy suite.

Histology Laboratory

We collected a task-based breathing zone air sample for formaldehyde on the histologist while she prepared, processed, and fixed tissue samples collected during autopsies. Area air samples were taken in the tissue preparation area and in the area next to the tissue processor during this same period (Table 2). Sampling times were approximately 75 minutes for each of the samples. The results were below the concentrations measured in the autopsy suite and did not exceed any short-term ceiling limits.

Table 2. Air sampling results for formaldehyde collected in the histology laboratory on January 11, 2012

Sample location	Sample type	Sampling period (minutes)	Concentration (ppm)
Histologist	PBZ	76	0.05
Tissue preparation	GA	75	0.01
Tissue processing	GA	74	0.01
NIOSH REL			C 0.1
ACGIH TLV			C 0.3

PBZ = personal breathing zone
GA = general area
C = ceiling

Chemicals containing organic compounds were used in the tissue processor. We collected area air samples to screen for a wide range of organic compounds that may have volatilized into the ambient work environment. Results of two screening samples showed low levels of branched C_8–C_{12} aliphatic hydrocarbons, ethanol, and isopropanol.

Fingerprint Evidence Laboratory

A task-based breathing zone air sample for ethyl 2-cyanoacrylate was taken on the latent fingerprint specialist during the processing of a piece of evidence. Three general area air samples were also taken in the area during this time (Table 3). Only the personal breathing zone sample returned a result (0.06 ppm) above the minimum quantifiable concentration (0.05 ppm). While no short-term occupational exposure limits (OELs) exist for ethyl

Table 3. Air sampling results for ethyl 2-cyanoacrylate collected on January 11, 2012

Sample location	Sample type	Sampling period (minutes)	Concentration (ppm)
Fingerprint developer	PBZ	56	0.06
Next to fuming chamber	GA	57	[0.05]*
Next to room door	GA	58	[0.04]
Outside fingerprint room	GA	59	ND

PBZ = personal breathing zone
GA = general area
C = ceiling
*Concentrations between the minimum detectable concentration and minimum quantifiable concentration are shown in brackets.

2-cyanoacrylate, ACGIH has set an 8-hour time-weighted average (TWA) threshold limit value (TLV) at 0.2 ppm.

Work practices in the fingerprint development room included evacuating vapors from the fuming chamber through an outlet on the side of the chamber. During the evacuation, a paper towel was draped over the outlet, and an adjacent ductless hood was turned on to capture emissions (Figure 7). This ductless hood was equipped with a high-efficiency particulate air filter. High-efficiency particulate air filters can capture particles successfully, but are not useful in removing vapors such as ethyl 2-cyanoacrylate. A carbon filter or combination carbon/high-efficiency particulate air filter would be needed to remove vapor phase contaminants such as ethyl 2-cyanoacrylate. Independent cyanoacrylate fume extractors that can be attached directly to the outlet of the fuming chamber are available commercially and can be used as an alternative, if desired.

Ventilation measurements were taken at each of the exhaust and supply vents within the fingerprint evidence laboratory room (Figure B2). The supply vents supplied 322 cfm of air to the room. The exhaust vent exhausted 474 cfm. Smoke tubes were used to generate small quantities of smoke at the doorway to the room to visualize air flow patterns. Measurements confirmed that the room was under negative pressure in relation to the adjacent room.

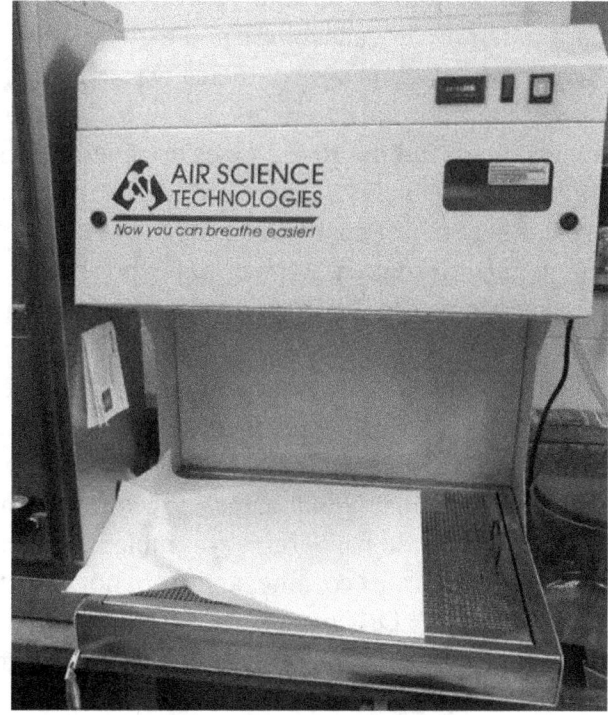

Figure 7. Ductless hood used during evacuation of vapors.

Table 4. Personal breathing zone and general area air concentrations of methamphetamine, cocaine, THC particles, and heroin measured in the drug evidence laboratory on January 12, 2012

Sample location	Sample type	Time (minutes)	Concentrations (ng/m^3)			
			Methamphetamine	Cocaine	THC	Heroin
Drug analyst 1	PBZ	55	140	ND	ND	1,900
Drug analyst 2	PBZ	112	60	ND	ND	190
Drug analyst 3	PBZ	90	63	200	1.4	2,900
On GC/MS 4	GA	174	38	ND	ND	120
On GC/MS 1	GA	174	12	ND	0.76	86
Drug storage vault	GA	173	ND	ND	ND	ND
Minimum detectable concentrations*			6–19	70–220	0.43–1.3	2.3–7.2

PBZ = personal breathing zone
GA = general area
THC = tetrahydrocannabinol
ND = not detected
GC/MS = gas chromatography/mass spectrometry
*Minimum detectable concentrations were established for each sample and varied on the basis of individual sample volumes.

Drug Evidence Laboratory

Personal breathing zone and general area air samples were collected and analyzed for cocaine, heroin, tetrahydrocannabinol, and methamphetamine. Specifically, a task-based breathing zone sample for airborne drug particles was collected on each of the three forensic drug analysts during their normal case work activities. During this sampling period, each forensic drug analyst analyzed the 10–12 cases assigned for the work shift. Because certain cases required multiple drug analyses, each forensic analyst analyzed 21–36 samples. This represented a typical quantity of analyses during a work shift. The time sampled represented the period during the work shift of greatest potential exposures to aerosolized drug particles. The forensic drug analysts do not do activities that require manipulation of drug samples during the rest of the shift. Three general area air samples were also collected during this period. Two of these were collected near the gas chromatography/mass spectrometry instruments in the drug evidence laboratory. The third was collected outside of the laboratory in the drug storage vault. Results are shown in Table 4. No OELs exist for the drugs we sampled. In a previous HHE at a police officer drug vault, similar sampling was conducted. Results from that evaluation ranged from not detected to 28 nanograms per cubic meter (ng/m^3) for methamphetamine, from not detected to 12,000 ng/m^3 for cocaine, and from not detected to > 54 ng/m^3 for tetrahydrocannabinol [NIOSH 2011]. Differences in concentrations compared to this previous evaluation may reflect the types of drugs with which the analysts worked. Heroin was described by each of the three forensic drug analysts sampled as the main drug analyzed during the sampling period. As in the previous NIOSH evaluation, personal breathing zone air concentrations were higher than area air concentrations.

Ten surface wipe samples for drug particles were collected in various areas of the drug evidence laboratory. The ten samples were collected in side-by-side pairs (as requested by the analytical laboratory) so that five locations were sampled (Figure B3). Three of the pairs were collected at the workstations of the three drug forensic scientists. One pair was collected next to a balance used to weigh samples in one of the work areas. The final pair was collected at a computer workstation to the left of gas chromatography/mass spectrometry 1 where no drug analysis work was done and where it was suggested that the likelihood of drug particle contamination would be less.

Wipe sample results are shown in Table 5. Currently, no criteria exist for hazardous levels of drug particle contamination on surfaces in the workplace. The highest surface concentration of drug particles was for cocaine. The highest concentrations were measured at 190,000 nanograms per square centimeter (ng/100 cm^2) for the pair of samples collected next to the balance across from chemical safety hood 2B. Surface concentrations of cocaine at the workstations where the three forensic drug analysts worked ranged from 1,600–82,000 ng/100 cm^2. Cocaine contamination at a concentration of 10,000–11,000 ng/100 cm^2 was found on the desk surface of the computer station to the left of gas chromatography/mass spectrometry 1, indicating possible migration of contamination because no drugs were analyzed on this desktop. For comparison, wipe sampling for cocaine in a previous HHE at a police officers' drug vault returned maximum concentrations of 7,300 ng/100 cm^2 [NIOSH 2011].

Table 5. Drugs on surfaces in the drug evidence laboratory on January 12, 2012

Sample location	Mass per area (ng/100 cm^2)			
	Methamphetamine	Cocaine	THC	Heroin
Next to balance across from hood 2B	3,200	190,000	ND	40,000
Next to balance across from hood 2B	2,200	190,000	ND	16,000
Workstation surface to the right of hood 2B	ND	82,000	ND	4,200
Workstation surface to the right of hood 2B	ND	9,600	ND	9,100
Workstation surface to the right of hood 2C	ND	16,000	ND	5,700
Workstation surface to the right of hood 2C	ND	7,400	ND	4,700
Workstation surface across from hood 1B	8,700	1,600	ND	5,300
Workstation surface across from hood 1B	9,600	4,600	ND	5,400
Computer workstation near GC/MS 1	1,300	10,000	ND	1,900
Computer workstation near GC/MS 1	ND	11,000	ND	1,400
Limits of detection*	390–2000	860–30,000	2.2	13–350

THC = tetrahydrocannabinol
ND = not detected
GC/MS = gas chromatography/mass spectrometry
*Limits of detection were established for each sample and varied on the basis of dilution factors. Higher drug concentrations on samples required dilution during analysis to achieve a response in the analytical range of the assay, resulting in higher limits of detection for those samples.

All heroin samples returned results above the limit of detection. Concentrations of heroin particles were also greatest at the sampling location next to the balance (16,000–40,000 ng/100 cm²). Concentrations in all other locations measured between 1,400 (at gas chromatography/mass spectrometry 1) and 9,100 ng/100 cm² (at a workstation of one of the drug forensic scientists).

Half of the methamphetamine samples returned results above the limit of detection. Methamphetamine concentrations were greatest at one of the scientist's workstations (8,700–9,600 ng/100 cm²) followed by the sample location next to the balance (2,200–3,200 ng/100 cm²). For comparison, wipe sampling for methamphetamine in a previous police officers' drug vault HHE returned maximum concentrations of 79 ng/100 cm² [NIOSH 2011].

Results of all wipe samples for tetrahydrocannabinol were below the limit of detection.

Ventilation measurements were taken at each of the exhaust and supply vents within the drug evidence laboratory as well as at face of each of the ducted fume hoods (Figure B3). The supply vents supplied 2,176 cfm of air to the laboratory. The exhaust vent and hoods exhausted 2,144 cfm. Measurements confirmed the laboratory was under approximately neutral pressure in relation to the adjacent room.

Firearms Section

A breathing zone sample for lead was taken on the firearms examiner who fired several weapons in the firing room and into the water tank. Two general area air samples for lead were taken in the firing room during shooting, and one was taken directly outside the firing room (Table 6). The highest concentration of lead was found in the breathing zone of the firearms examiner at 100 μg/m³. The concentration of lead in both general area air samples collected in the firing room while shooting were similar: 37 μg/m³ near the bullet trap and 44 μg/m³ near the door. The door to the firing room was kept closed during the weapons firing, which likely explains why the concentration of lead collected by the general area air sample in the anteroom outside the firing room was below the minimum quantifiable concentration during shooting. There is no short-term or ceiling OEL for lead to directly

Table 6. Air sampling results for lead collected on January 12, 2012

Sample location	Sample type	Sampling period (minutes)	Concentration (μg/m³)
Firearms examiner	PBZ	60	100
Near bullet trap	GA	60	37
Near back wall next to firing room door	GA	62	44
Outside room	GA	60	[2.0]*

PBZ = personal breathing zone
GA = general area
*Concentrations between the minimum detectable concentration and minimum quantifiable concentration are shown in brackets.

compare these results. If the firearms examiner were to continue these same activities throughout the shift, the exposure to lead at this concentration could exceed full-shift OELs including the OSHA permissible exposure limit (PEL) and the NIOSH recommended exposure limit (REL), both set at 50 $\mu g/m^3$.

Nine surface wipe samples were collected for lead. One of these samples was collected on the hands of the firearms examiner after he fired weapons. Several were collected on floors and work surfaces inside and outside the firing room (Figure B4). Two were collected on surfaces on or around the water tank. Results of lead wipe samples are shown in Table 7. Not surprisingly, the highest concentration of lead was found on the floor in front of the bullet trap at 750 $\mu g/100$ cm^2. The next highest concentration (380

Table 7. Surface sampling results for lead collected on January 12, 2012

Sample location	Mass per area ($\mu g/100$ cm^2)
Firearms examiner's hands	120*
Water tank surface	37
Water tank floor	23
Range floor near door	20
Range floor where fired	25
Range floor next to bullet trap	750
Range bench top	380
Desk surface in anteroom	[1.3]†
Anteroom floor near far door	4.9

*The sample was wiped from the firearms examiner's hands and does not represent a 100-square-centimeter measured area.

†Concentrations between the minimum detectable concentration and minimum quantifiable concentration are shown in brackets.

$\mu g/100$ cm^2) was found on the bench top on the right hand side of the firing room. The result of wiping the hands of the firearms examiner after firing revealed 120 μg of lead. The result for the surface of a desk in the firing room's anteroom was below the minimum quantifiable concentration. No criteria exist for lead contamination on surfaces in the workplace. However, the presence of lead indicates a need for improved controls and administrative practices.

The firing room had a supply vent in the ceiling at the far end of the room near the bullet trap and an exhaust vent in the ceiling near the door. The exhaust vent was controlled by a switch in the firing room near the door. Standard practice during firings was to close the door between the firing room and the adjacent anteroom and to turn on the exhaust fan. The door was opened and the exhaust fan was turned off when firings were not occurring. Ventilation measurements were taken at the exhaust and supply vents within the firing room (Figure B4). The supply vent supplied 492 cfm of air to the room. When turned on, the exhaust vent exhausted 553 cfm of air. Smoke tubes were used to generate small quantities of smoke at points in the firing room to visualize airflow patterns. When the exhaust was turned on, smoke tube testing at the door showed no airflow in or out of the room; therefore, the room was under neutral pressure relative to the adjacent anteroom. Additionally, because of the configuration of the supply vent near the bullet trap and exhaust vent near the door, air did not flow from the point where the weapons were fired away from the firearms examiner toward the bullet trap as is recommended for firing ranges. When the exhaust was turned off, the room was under positive pressure relative to the adjacent anteroom, meaning air flowed from the firing room to the anteroom.

Discussion

Employees in the coroner's office autopsy suites faced a number of occupational hazards inherent to their work. These included potential exposures to infectious agents because of the procedures performed and the population being assessed [CDC 2012]. All autopsies involve potential exposures to blood and other body fluids, a risk of being splashed or splattered upon, and a risk of percutaneous injury [Nolte et al. 2002]. In fact, employee interviews and injury record reviews identified at least four needlestick and two scalpel injuries in the past few years. Exposure to sharp objects within the body and bone fragments may also result in cuts, and the manipulation of large organs may result in body splashes [CDC 2012]. During these procedures, autopsy suite employees may be at risk of exposure to infectious agents such as *Mycobacterium tuberculosis* and bloodborne pathogens such as Hepatitis B and C, and human immunodeficiency virus [Nolte et al. 2002].

Procedures that involve the use of oscillating saws may create airborne particles that contain infectious pathogens such as *Mycobacterium tuberculosis* as well as those not normally transmitted by the inhalation route; such particles can also contaminate inanimate surfaces [Nolte et al. 2002]. A procedure that potentially generates high concentrations of infectious aerosols is skull cap removal [Green and Yoshida 1990]. Droplets of blood and cerebrospinal fluid as well as the interstices of bone matrix may contain these infectious agents, but they could also be carried on the surface of particles formed by the combination of bone dust particles with fluid droplets [Green and Yoshida 1990]. The median diameter of bone dust particles in the breathing zone of a saw operator generated during a cranial autopsy has been reported to be 0.37 µm, which can remain airborne for long periods of time, be inhaled, and easily penetrate the alveolar region of the lung [Green and Yoshida 1990]. No local exhaust ventilation was used with the oscillating saw.

Past NIOSH evaluations of cranial autopsies with and without the aid of local exhaust ventilation indicate that the use of local exhaust ventilation had a significant effect on reducing the aerosols produced by the saws [NIOSH 1997]. Our data also indicate that peaks in aerosol concentrations were produced during use of the oscillating saw in the autopsy suite. The highest peaks were observed during the use of the saw at the autopsy table under the aerosol monitor. We observed only one small peak during the times of saw use at the far autopsy table, approximately 10–15 feet away. Given the distance, this suggests that air mixing in the room was limited and the greatest potential for employee exposures occurred at the table where they were removing the skull cap. Capture of the aerosols produced by the saw through local exhaust ventilation would assist in reducing the potential for exposure of saw operators to infectious aerosols. We observed an autopsy employee handling the oscillating saw to remove skull caps while wearing a surgical mask, which does not provide respiratory protection. A NIOSH-approved N95 respirator is the minimum recommended level of respiratory protection for work in autopsy suites [CDC 2012].

Formaldehyde, as a component of formalin used for specimen preservation, is the most common chemical to which autopsy employees are exposed [CDC 2012]. The most commonly reported health complaints due to exposure to low concentrations of formaldehyde include irritation of the eyes, nose, and throat; nasal congestion; headaches; skin rash; and asthma [NRC 1981]. It is often difficult to attribute specific health effects to particular concentrations of formaldehyde because some people may have symptoms at levels where others may experience no symptoms [NRC 1981]. Most employees did not report such symptoms during the medical interviews, with the exception of headaches being reported by two employees. The work-relatedness of these could not be determined.

Formaldehyde concentrations during short-term sampling periods during autopsies ranged from 0.10–0.46 ppm. All short-term samples returned results that were at or above the ceiling limit of 0.1 ppm recommended by NIOSH, with one result above the ceiling limit of 0.3 ppm recommended by ACGIH. Sample results were not calculated for full work shift exposures but may have exceeded the NIOSH full-shift REL of 0.016 ppm. However, this full-shift REL was established in 1981 when NIOSH first recognized formaldehyde as a potential occupational carcinogen. On the basis of the carcinogen policy in existence at the time, NIOSH set the REL to the "lowest feasible concentration," which for formaldehyde was defined as the analytical limit of quantification of 0.016 ppm for up to a 10-hour TWA and a ceiling limit of 0.10 ppm that should not be exceeded [NIOSH 1981]. However, research has shown that concentrations of formaldehyde in ambient air can approach or exceed this level [Lemen 1987]. Additionally, the subsequent revision of the NIOSH carcinogen policy [NIOSH 1995], combined with better exposure characterization and advances in risk assessment and management strategies, support the need for NIOSH to reassess the formaldehyde REL.

On the basis of the exhaust measurements and the measured dimensions of the autopsy suite, the calculated number of air changes per hour for the room was 5.4. This is below the recommended 12 air changes per hour for autopsy rooms. However, this calculated number of air changes per hour for this room is likely an underestimation. Smoke tube testing identified a considerable pressure differential between the autopsy room and the adjacent main cooler room, which had a garage-type roll-up door that opened between them. This cooler room was one location where bodies were stored before and after autopsies. Although this door closed during autopsies, we observed that air from the autopsy room was pulled around the edges of the closed door into the main cooler room as a result of an exhaust fan operating in the main cooler room. The main cooler room was under greater negative pressure. Therefore, air from the autopsy room was also exhausted through the cooler room in addition to the exhaust vents. Nevertheless, improved ventilation exhaust rates in the autopsy room are recommended. One way to increase exhaust is to use downdraft tables that provide local exhaust ventilation at the table level. NIOSH has researched the use of local exhaust ventilation to reduce formaldehyde exposures during embalming procedures [Gressel and Hughes 1992]. Because of its effectiveness in reducing formaldehyde exposures, NIOSH recommended using this type of local exhaust ventilation as a primary exposure control rather than increasing the general room (dilution) ventilation. It was determined that, depending on how well the air in the room is mixed, 4–13 times more general dilution exhaust air would be needed to achieve the same control as from the local exhaust ventilation system at the embalming table [NIOSH 1998a]. Reducing the time formalin-containing jars are open is also important in minimizing formaldehyde exposures in the autopsy suite.

Work processes in the histology lab required opening formalin-containing tissue specimen jars to prepare specimens for mounting on slides. Formaldehyde sampling during these processes revealed lower airborne formaldehyde concentrations than those in the autopsy suite, ranging from 0.01–0.05 ppm. This may be due to a number of factors including the presence of an exhaust hood where the histologist opened the specimen jars and the shorter periods for which the formalin-containing jars remained opened in the histology laboratory compared to the autopsy suite.

Similar to practices observed in the autopsy suites, drug forensic scientists did not use disposable safety scalpels or blade removal devices. The drug section employees should use particular caution while cutting pills and substances for analysis and when handling hypodermic needles. Exposures to airborne drug particles were present, but appeared to be low. Despite this, repeated exposures may present a health hazard, even at low concentrations and through routes that are not typical for these drugs. Additionally, the possibility of unknown interactions with drug or prescription medication can be a concern. No OELs exist for comparing these airborne concentrations. However, concentrations were roughly in the same ranges as in a past HHE of a police officers' drug vault, with personal breathing zone air concentrations of methamphetamine being slightly higher, while concentrations of cocaine and tetrahydrocannabinol were lower. Le et al. [1992] reported airborne cocaine concentrations as high as 6,400,000 ng/m^3 during sampling of criminalists during simulations of field situations in which the contents of 25 or 50 one-kilo packages of cocaine were transferred. The study emphasized the need to use caution, particularly during work on large cocaine-seizure cases, and suggested limiting the generation of airborne cocaine dust to reduce the levels of exposure [Le et al. 1992].

Also of concern was evidence of contamination of work surfaces with drug particles. While there are no criteria for comparison, it is wise to reduce exposure to all drug particles as much as feasible. Particles can be transferred from surfaces to hands, and in the absence of adequate hand washing, can then be transferred from hands to mouth or eyes, representing a possible route of exposure to the drugs. No federal standards exist for drug surface contamination; however several states have established feasibility-based surface contamination limits when remediating clandestine laboratories for methamphetamine. These range from $\leq$ 100 ng/100 cm^2 to 500 ng/100 cm^2 [NAMSDL 2008]. Results of surface sampling in the drug evidence laboratory for methamphetamine ranged up to 9,600 ng/100 cm^2.

Firearms examiners are exposed to lead and occupational noise in the course of their job tasks. Air sampling during shooting identified the possibility of high levels of lead exposure to the firearms examiner. During the 60 minutes we sampled, only five gunshots were fired, but they resulted in a high concentration of airborne lead. The concentration of airborne lead produced by these few shots was high enough that exposures could have exceeded full-shift occupational limits if similar shooting activities had continued throughout the 8-hour shift. Description of work practices provided by the firearms examiners indicated that shooting at that frequency consistently throughout an 8-hour shift was not a typical occurrence. However, it was noted that some days did require multiple weapons firings throughout the day to process a heavy case load. In these instances, lead exposure is a concern and further evaluation of full shift exposures is warranted. Surface sampling, particularly around the area of the bullet trap and on the bench tops of the firing room, identified the need to improve cleaning and maintenance practices to avoid dermal contamination and hand-to-mouth transmission of lead which may lead to ingestion. The current ventilation configuration may have pulled lead-contaminated air through the employee's breathing zone instead of away from it.

Noise-induced hearing loss is one of the most common occupational diseases [NIOSH 2001]. Although we did not monitor noise exposures during the evaluation, the firearms examiners were exposed to impulsive noise when firing weapons. While their exposures were typically short, prolonged exposures to impulse noise may lead to noise-induced hearing loss [Chan et al. 2001]. Individual employees' annual audiograms were compared to their baseline audiogram to determine if a standard threshold shift had occurred. OSHA states that a standard threshold shift is a change in hearing threshold, relative to the baseline audiogram, of an average of 10 decibels or more at 2,000, 3,000, and 4,000 hertz in one or both ears [29 CFR 1904.10; 29 CFR 1910.95]. The NIOSH-recommended threshold shift criterion is a 15 decibel shift at any frequency from 500–6000 hertz in either ear measured twice in succession [NIOSH 1998b]. The firearms examiners had neither an OSHA standard threshold shift nor a NIOSH threshold shift on their 5-year follow-up audiograms compared to their baseline audiograms in either ear.

Conclusions

Most interviewed employees expressed workplace-related concerns, including concerns about building ventilation and potential chemical exposures. Additionally, they mentioned overcrowding and insufficient workspace, and we observed equipment stored or used in rooms or halls where they were not originally intended to be used. We also observed boxes and equipment stored in locations such as in front of autopsy suite exhaust vents, which may have affected the potential for exposures because of their impact on ventilation airflow. A small number of employees reported headaches and stress as symptoms they felt were work-related although we were not able to assess the work-relatedness of these symptoms. Self-reports of injuries mainly involved those incurred from needlesticks and scalpel blades. Task-based sampling for formaldehyde in the autopsy suite identified results at or above recommended ceiling limits, suggesting that further controls were necessary to reduce this hazard. Additionally, observations of work practices in the autopsy suite identified the need for improved use of personal protective equipment and additional controls (practices, devices, or both) to help reduce the possibility of sharps injuries. Task-based air sampling for drug particles showed the presence of aerosolized drugs in the breathing zone of analysts as they analyzed drugs. Surface sampling showed that drug particle contamination in the drug evidence laboratory and lead contamination in the firing room were potential hazards. Air sampling for lead indicated that airborne lead exposures could pose a hazard if weapons were fired throughout a work shift at the rate observed during sampling. Implementing the recommendations below will help limit exposures and reduce occupational hazards. Future facility changes should involve the input of employees and should use a prevention-through-design approach, a concept in which occupational injuries and illnesses are prevented and controlled by "designing out" or minimizing the hazards and risks early in the design process [Howard 2008].

Recommendations

On the basis of our findings, we recommend the actions listed below. We encourage the coroner's office to use a labor-management health and safety committee or working group to discuss our recommendations and develop an action plan. Those involved in the work can best set priorities and assess the feasibility of our recommendations for the specific situation at the coroner's office.

Our recommendations are based on an approach known as the hierarchy of controls (Appendix C). This approach groups actions by their likely effectiveness in reducing or removing hazards. In most cases, the preferred approach is to eliminate hazardous materials or processes and install engineering controls to reduce exposure or shield employees. Until such controls are in place, or if they are not effective or feasible, administrative measures and personal protective equipment may be needed.

Engineering Controls

Engineering controls reduce exposures to employees by removing the hazard from the process or placing a barrier between the hazard and the employee. Engineering controls are very effective at protecting employees without placing primary responsibility of implementation on the employee.

1. Increase the number of air changes per hour in the autopsy suite.
2. Use downdraft tables that are exhausted outside to capture airborne contaminants such as formaldehyde originating from the autopsy work processes at their source or point of generation.
3. Use local exhaust ventilation attachments when using the saw for cranial autopsies.
4. Modify the existing supply and exhaust ventilation in the firing room to provide a laminar flow of air that passes from the shooter toward the bullet trap. Ensure that slightly more air is exhausted than supplied to maintain appropriate negative pressure in the firing room [NIOSH 2009]. In the interim, limit the number of weapons tested in one day.
5. Use high-efficiency particulate air filtered hoods for work processes during which drug particles may become aerosolized.
6. Install a carbon filter or combination carbon/high-efficiency particulate air filter for the ductless hood adjacent to the fuming chamber, or use an independent cyanoacrylate fume extractor that can be directly attached to the outlet of the fuming chamber during evacuation of the fingerprint development chamber.

Administrative Controls

The term administrative controls refers to employer-dictated work practices and policies to reduce or prevent hazardous exposures. Their effectiveness depends on employer commitment and employee acceptance. Regular monitoring and reinforcement are necessary to ensure that policies and procedures are followed consistently.

1. Replace lids on containers of formaldehyde as soon as possible after use.
2. Improve cleaning practices in the drug evidence laboratory to remove drug particles on work surfaces. Use either a high-efficiency particulate air filtered vacuum or wet cleaning techniques with detergent and water to clean nonporous surfaces. Eliminating porous surfaces, joints, and crevices is also recommended.
3. Improve cleaning practices in the firing room to clean up lead contamination on floor and work surfaces. Do not dry sweep in the firing room; use a high-efficiency particulate air filtered vacuum or wet mopping methods. Use mops and cleaning tools that are dedicated to this activity. The OSHA general industry lead standard states that shoveling, dry or wet sweeping, and brushing may be used only where vacuuming or other equally effective methods have been tried and found ineffective [29 CFR 1910.1025].
4. Do full-shift monitoring periodically for lead exposures in the firing range on days when multiple firearm shootings will be performed consistently throughout the shift.
5. Do periodic short-term and full-shift follow-up monitoring for formaldehyde in the autopsy suite.
6. Advise all shooters to wash their hands thoroughly after firing weapons. Provide soap or wipes that have been formulated specifically to remove lead from the skin.
7. Wash hands before leaving the autopsy suite. After noticing a glove puncture, wash hands immediately with soap and water before resuming the autopsy. Consider all surfaces to be potentially contaminated.
8. Use disposable safety scalpels. However, if reusable scalpels are used, then use scalpel blade removal devices rather than removing blades manually [Perry et al. 2003].
9. Instruct employees to hold skin flaps with forceps and not with the hands when suturing with string or other suture materials at the end of an autopsy on the skull cap, chest cavity, or other part of the body.
10. Use a test tube rack to hold test tubes while filling them with blood, vitreous fluid, or urine samples rather than holding the test tube itself to help prevent accidental needlesticks.
11. Ensure sharps containers are not filled greater than two-thirds full. When two-thirds full, close and dispose of the container properly and replace it with a new container.
12. Move items such as trash cans, boxes, and equipment from in front of exhaust vents in the autopsy suite, and do not use these locations for storage.
13. Use a colorimetric wipe method periodically to disclose the presence of lead on skin surfaces as a part of health and safety training. This method allows direct and timely observation of contamination by lead and allows shooters to see that evidence on their hands.

14. Continue audiometric testing to compare to baseline levels upon initial assignment in a noisy work area and at the time of reassignment out of the area. Audiograms should be done annually as long as the employee is assigned to a job where the TWA exposure level is equal to or greater than 85 A-weighted decibels. If an audiogram indicates a standard threshold shift, refer the employee for a medical evaluation.
15. Provide employees access to their records upon request, and review medical tests such as audiograms and BLLs with employees.

Personal Protective Equipment

Personal protective equipment is the least effective means for controlling hazardous exposures. Proper use of personal protective equipment requires a comprehensive program and requires a high level of employee involvement and commitment. The right personal protective equipment must be chosen for each hazard. Supporting programs such as training, change-out schedules, and medical assessment may be needed. Personal protective equipment should not be the sole method for controlling hazardous exposures. Rather, personal protective equipment should be used until effective engineering and administrative controls are in place.

1. Require, at a minimum, NIOSH-approved N95 filtering facepiece respirators for employees in the autopsy suite [CDC 2012]. Surgical masks do not protect autopsy personnel from inhaling airborne particles. A respiratory protection program as defined in the OSHA respiratory protection standard [29 CFR 1910.134] should be implemented. If personnel are unable to wear a NIOSH-approved N95 negative pressure respirator because of facial hair or other limitation, then they should wear a NIOSH-approved loose-fitting powered air purifying respirator with high efficiency filters.
2. Use the following additional personal protective equipment during autopsies: fluid-resistant apron and sleeves; booties; surgical caps; and eye and face protection such as goggles and a transparent shield that covers the face, mouth, and neck (unless a powered air purifying respirator is worn). Eyeglasses alone are not adequate protection. Use double gloves and change both gloves every hour. Select a cut-resistant glove of fine-woven steel to prevent cuts from bone and scalpels, and cover with a rubber glove for slip resistance. These gloves do not protect against needlesticks [CDC 2012].
3. Wear protective safety goggles that prevent exposure to splashes from formaldehyde or other chemicals while fixing tissues in the histology laboratory.
4. Wear lab coats and safety glasses during work in the drug evidence laboratory.
5. Use double hearing protection (earmuffs and ear plugs) for impulsive noise generated during weapons firing [NIOSH 2009].

Appendix A: Methods

Formaldehyde

Personal breathing zone and general area air samples for formaldehyde were collected on 2,4-dinitrophenylhydrazine-treated silica gel cartridges. Tygon® tubing connecting the sampler and sampling pump allowed air to be drawn at a calibrated flow rate of 50 milliliters per minute and 200 milliliters per minute, depending on the anticipated sampling time. For personal breathing zone air samples, the sampling media was attached to the employee's lapel within the breathing zone, roughly defined as an area in front of the shoulders with a radius of 6 to 9 inches. Analysis of the cartridges was performed according to NIOSH Method 2016, with modifications [NIOSH 2010a]. The limit of detection was 0.02 micrograms (µg) formaldehyde per sample, and the limit of quantitation was 0.051 µg formaldehyde/sample.

Air Sampling for Lead

Personal breathing zone and general area air samples for lead were collected on 37-millimeter diameter, 0.8-µm pore size mixed cellulose ester filters using Aircheck 2000S air sampling pumps (SKC, Inc, Eighty Four, Pennsylvania) calibrated at a flow rate of 2 liters per minute. The inlet port of the sampling pump was connected to the sampling media with Tygon® tubing. For personal breathing zone air samples, the sampling media was attached to the employee's lapel within the breathing zone. Air samples were analyzed using inductively coupled plasma according to NIOSH Method 7303 [NIOSH 2010a]. The limit of detection was 0.2 µg/sample, and the limit of quantitation was 0.55 µg/sample.

Surface Wipe Sampling for Lead

Surface wipe samples were collected with premoistened Wash n' Dri wipes (Colgate USA, New York). The collection procedure was as follows: (1) identify the area to be sampled; (2) put on a pair of gloves; (3) place the wipe flat on the surface as defined by the 10 centimeter × 10 centimeter (100-square-centimeter area) disposable template and wipe the surface using three to four vertical S-strokes, side-to-side so that the entire surface is covered; (4) fold the exposed side of the wipe in and wipe the area with three or four horizontal S-strokes; (5) fold the wipe once more and wipe the area with three or four vertical S-strokes; and (6) fold the pad, exposed side in, and place in a sterile container. A new template and a pair of disposable gloves were used for each surface wipe sample. The surface wipe samples were digested and analyzed by inductively coupled argon plasma-atomic emission spectroscopy according to NIOSH Method 9102 [NIOSH 2010a]. The limit of detection was 0.4 µg/sample, and the limit of quantitation was 1.5 µg/sample.

Volatile Organic Compounds

Personal breathing zone and general area air sampling for volatile organic compounds used thermal desorption tubes attached to SKC pocket pumps calibrated at 200 milliliters per minute (SKC Inc., Eighty Four, Pennsylvania). The thermal desorption tubes contained three beds of sorbent material: (1) 90 milligrams of Carbopack™ Y, (2) 115 milligrams of Carbopack B, and (3) 150 milligrams Carboxen™. For personal breathing zone air samples, the sampling media was attached to the employee's lapel within the breathing zone. After sampling, the thermal desorption tubes were stored in a cooler and then qualitatively analyzed for volatile organic compounds according to NIOSH Method 2549 [NIOSH 2010a].

Air and Surface Sampling for Drugs

Personal breathing zone and general area air sampling for particle phase drugs was conducted using SKC 37-millimeter diameter, 2-μm pore size polytetrafluoroethylene filters attached to SKC Aircheck XR5000S pumps calibrated at 4 liters per minute. For personal breathing zone air samples, the sampling media was attached to the employee's lapel within the breathing zone. Surface sampling for drugs used cotton wipes pre-moistened with surface sampling buffer. For most sampling locations, a 10 centimeter × 10 centimeter template was placed over the surface and wiped using the pre-moistened cotton wipe in the same manner as surface wipe sampling for lead.

After sampling, the polytetrafluoroethylene filters and wipes were stored in a cooler and then analyzed for methamphetamine, heroin, cocaine, and tetrahydrocannabinol with a fluorescence covalent microbead immunosorbent assay as described by Smith et al. [2010]. A standard curve for each drug was generated to calculate equivalent values. The values of the drugs collected from the surfaces were corrected using the surface recovery values determined previously [Smith et al. 2010]. For the air samples, extraction was done in methanol; the extraction solutions were then dried, and the residue was re-extracted with the surface sampling buffer. The detection and quantitation limits were provided for each analyte. However, because trace drugs (or interfering compounds) were identified on the field and laboratory blanks, the detection limits were adjusted. Adjustments were made by adding the average analyte concentration measured on the field or laboratory blank (whichever was higher) to the respective detection limits.

Ethyl 2-Cyanoacrylate

Personal breathing zone and general area air samples were collected by drawing a flow rate of 100 milliliters per minute through the phosphoric acid-treated XAD-7 sampling tubes. For personal breathing zone air samples, the sampling media was attached to the employee's lapel within the breathing zone. Following desorption of the sample with 2 milliliters of 0.2% phosphoric acid in acetonitrile, the samples were analyzed by high pressure liquid chromatography with ultraviolet detection according to OSHA Method 55 [OSHA 1985].

Appendix B: Diagrams of Four Coroner's Office Sections

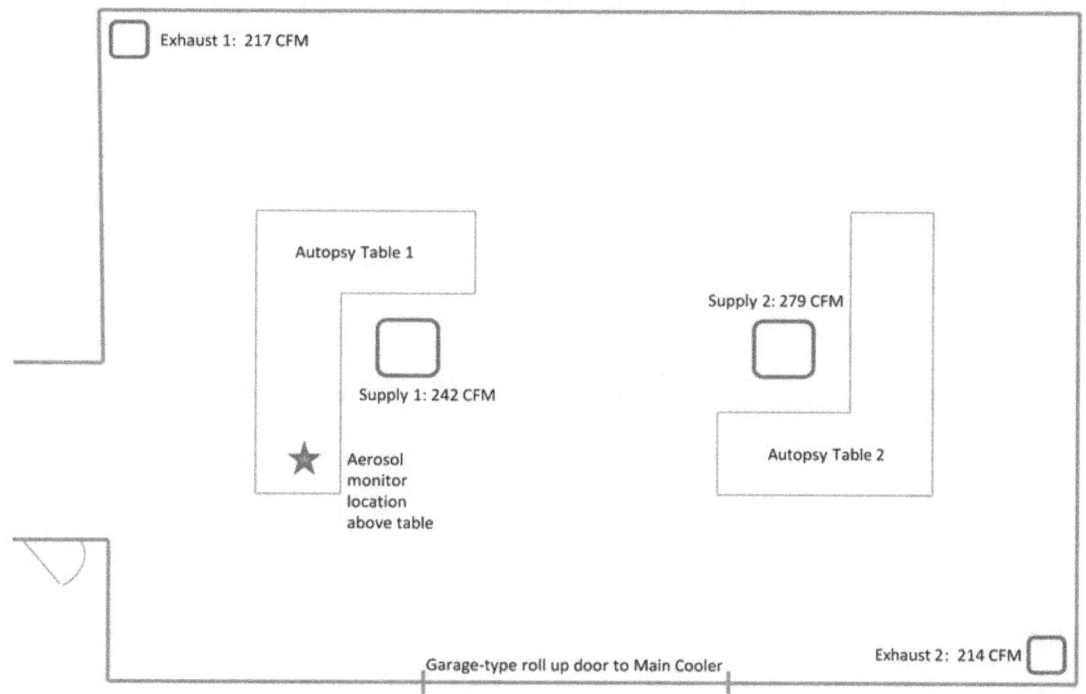

Figure B1. Diagram of ventilation measurements and the aerosol monitor location in autopsy suite 1.

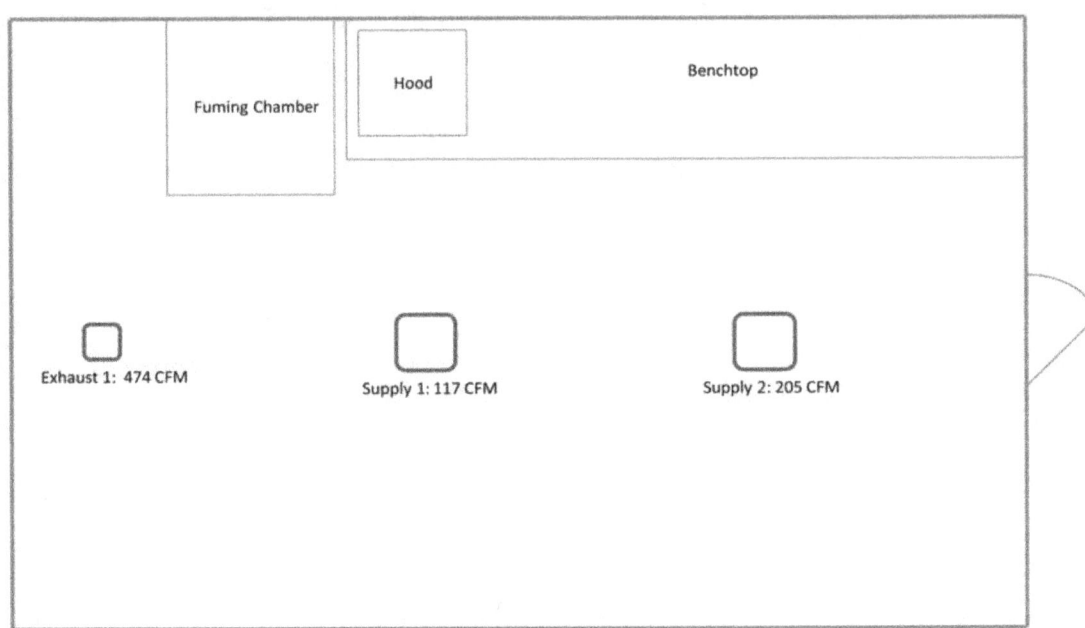

Figure B2. Diagram of ventilation measurements in the fingerprint evidence laboratory room.

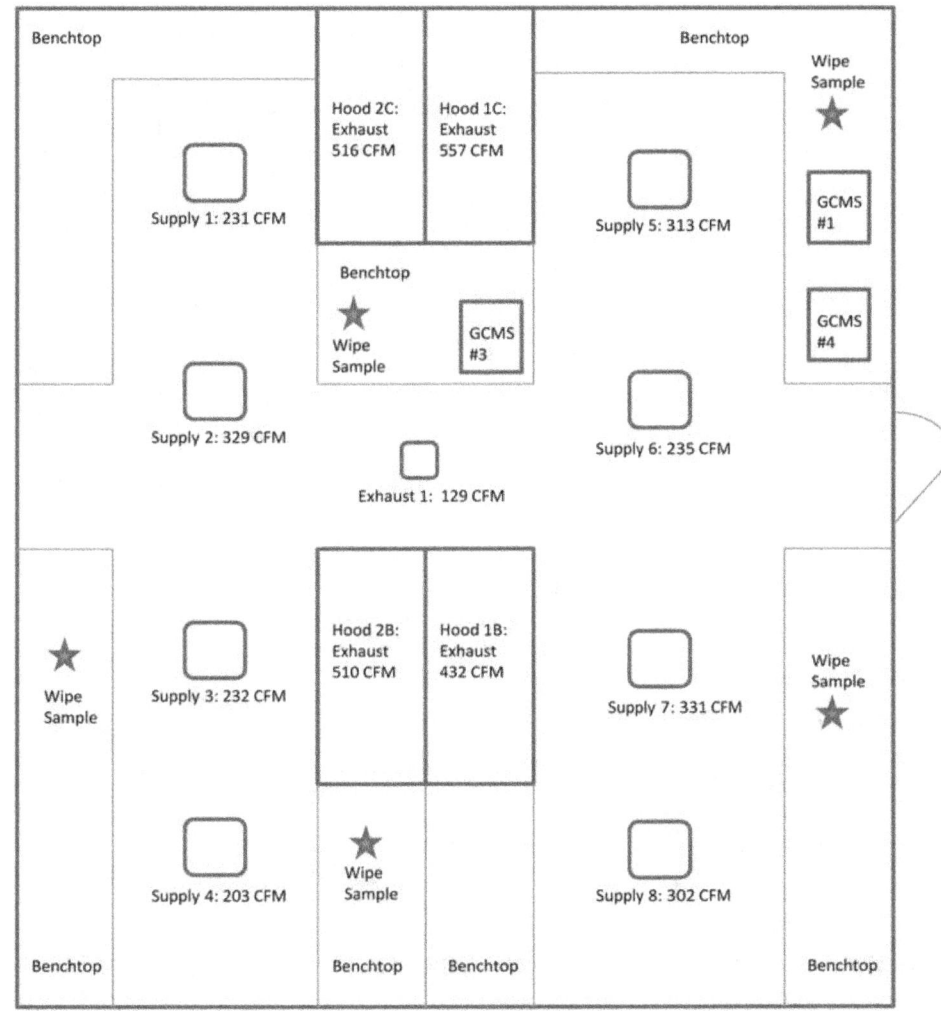

Figure B3. Diagram of ventilation measurements and wipe sample locations in the drug evidence laboratory.

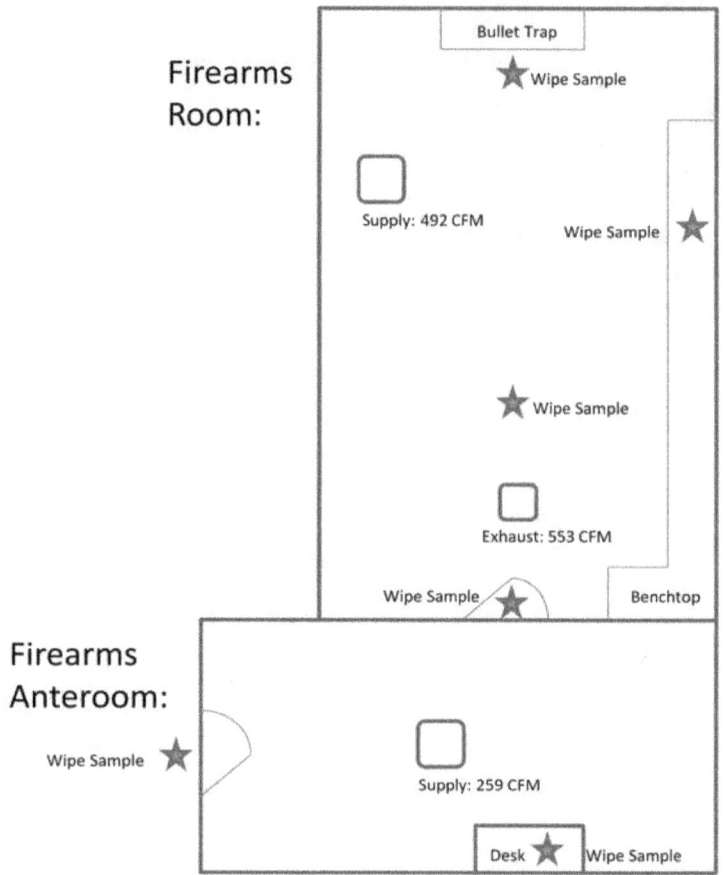

Figure B4. Diagram of ventilation measurements and wipe sample locations in the firearms section.

Appendix C: Occupational Exposure Limits and Health Effects

NIOSH investigators refer to mandatory (legally enforceable) and recommended OELs for chemical, physical, and biological agents when evaluating workplace hazards. OELs have been developed by federal agencies and safety and health organizations to prevent adverse health effects from workplace exposures. Generally, OELs suggest levels of exposure that most employees may be exposed to for up to 10 hours per day, 40 hours per week, for a working lifetime, without experiencing adverse health effects. However, not all employees will be protected if their exposures are maintained below these levels. Some may have adverse health effects because of individual susceptibility, a preexisting medical condition, or a hypersensitivity (allergy). In addition, some hazardous substances act in combination with other exposures, with the general environment, or with medications or personal habits of the employee to produce adverse health effects. Most OELs address airborne exposures. But, some substances can be absorbed directly through the skin and mucous membranes.

Most OELs are expressed as a TWA exposure. A TWA refers to the average exposure during a normal 8- to 10-hour workday. Some chemical substances and physical agents have recommended short-term exposure limit (STEL) or ceiling values. Unless otherwise noted, the short-term exposure limit is a 15-minute TWA exposure. It should not be exceeded at any time during a workday. The ceiling limit should not be exceeded at any time.

In the United States, OELs have been established by federal agencies, professional organizations, state and local governments, and other entities. Some OELs are legally enforceable limits; others are recommendations.

- The U.S. Department of Labor OSHA PELs (29 CFR 1910 [general industry]; 29 CFR 1926 [construction industry]; and 29 CFR 1917 [maritime industry]) are legal limits. These limits are enforceable in workplaces covered under the Occupational Safety and Health Act of 1970.

- NIOSH RELs are recommendations based on a critical review of the scientific and technical information and the adequacy of methods to identify and control the hazard. NIOSH RELs are published in the NIOSH Pocket Guide to Chemical Hazards [NIOSH 2010b]. NIOSH also recommends risk management practices (e.g., engineering controls, safe work practices, employee education/training, personal protective equipment, and exposure and medical monitoring) to minimize the risk of exposure and adverse health effects.

- Other OELs commonly used and cited in the United States include (a) the TLVs, which are recommended by ACGIH, a professional organization, and (b) the workplace environmental exposure levels (WEELs), which are recommended by the American Industrial Hygiene Association, another professional organization. The TLVs and

WEELs are developed by committee members of these associations from a review of the published, peer-reviewed literature. These OELs are not consensus standards. TLVs are considered voluntary exposure guidelines for use by industrial hygienists and others trained in this discipline "to assist in the control of health hazards" [ACGIH 2012]. WEELs have been established for some chemicals "when no other legal or authoritative limits exist" [AIHA 2012].

Outside the United States, OELs have been established by various agencies and organizations and include legal and recommended limits. The Institut für Arbeitsschutz der Deutschen Gesetzlichen Unfallversicherung (IFA, Institute for Occupational Safety and Health of the German Social Accident Insurance) maintains a database of international OELs from European Union member states, Canada (Québec), Japan, Switzerland, and the United States. The database, available at http://www.dguv.de/ifa/en/gestis/limit_values/index.jsp, contains international limits for more than 1,500 hazardous substances and is updated periodically.

OSHA requires an employer to furnish employees a place of employment free from recognized hazards that cause or are likely to cause death or serious physical harm [Occupational Safety and Health Act of 1970 (Public Law 91–596, sec. 5(a)(1))]. This is true in the absence of a specific OEL. It also is important to keep in mind that OELs may not reflect current health-based information.

When multiple OELs exist for a substance or agent, NIOSH investigators generally encourage employers to use the lowest OEL when making risk assessment and risk management decisions. NIOSH investigators also encourage use of the hierarchy of controls approach to eliminate or minimize workplace hazards. This includes, in order of preference, the use of (1) substitution or elimination of the hazardous agent, (2) engineering controls (e.g., local exhaust ventilation, process enclosure, dilution ventilation), (3) administrative controls (e.g., limiting time of exposure, employee training, work practice changes, medical surveillance), and (4) personal protective equipment (e.g., respiratory protection, gloves, eye protection, hearing protection). Control banding, a qualitative risk assessment and risk management tool, is a complementary approach to protecting employee health. Control banding focuses on how broad categories of risk should be managed. Information on control banding is available at http://www.cdc.gov/niosh/topics/ctrlbanding/. This approach can be applied in situations where OELs have not been established or can be used to supplement existing OELs.

Below we provide the OELs and surface contamination limits for the compounds we measured, as well as a discussion of the potential health effects from exposure to these compounds.

Formaldehyde

Under the OSHA general industry standard for airborne exposure to formaldehyde [29 CFR 1910.1048], the PEL is 0.75 ppm for an 8-hour TWA, the action level is 0.5 ppm for an 8-hour TWA, and the short-term exposure limit is 2 ppm for a 15-minute TWA. The standard requires medical surveillance for employees exposed to formaldehyde at or above the action level or short-term exposure limit.

The NIOSH REL for formaldehyde is 0.016 ppm for up to an 8-hour TWA. NIOSH also has a 15-minute ceiling limit of 0.1 ppm that is not to be exceeded during a work shift [NIOSH 2010b]. NIOSH recognized formaldehyde as a potential occupational carcinogen in 1981 and, following the NIOSH carcinogen policy in existence at the time, set the REL to the "lowest feasible concentration," which for formaldehyde was defined as the analytical limit of quantification of 0.016 ppm for up to 8 hours [NIOSH 1981]. Since then, experience has shown that this REL is actually not the "lowest feasible concentration" because formaldehyde in the ambient air can exceed 0.016 ppm, a fact later acknowledged by NIOSH [Lemen 1987]. Additionally, the subsequent revision of the NIOSH carcinogen policy [NIOSH 1995], combined with better exposure characterization and advances in risk assessment and management strategies, support the need for NIOSH to reassess the formaldehyde REL. This effort is in progress.

ACGIH lists formaldehyde as a sensitizer with a ceiling limit of 0.3 ppm [ACGIH 2012]. An ACGIH ceiling limit is an exposure that should not be exceeded at any time during the work shift.

The International Agency for Research on Cancer classifies formaldehyde as a human carcinogen (group 1) on the basis of associations between formaldehyde exposure and nasopharyngeal cancer and leukemia [Baan et al. 2009]. NIOSH considers formaldehyde as a potential occupational carcinogen, ACGIH lists formaldehyde as a suspected human carcinogen, and the U.S. Department of Health and Human Services lists formaldehyde as reasonably anticipated to be a human carcinogen in its 11th report on carcinogens [NIOSH 1981; DHHS 2011; ACGIH 2012].

Lead

Lead is ubiquitous in U.S. urban environments because of the widespread use of lead compounds in industry, gasoline, and paints during the past century. Exposure to lead occurs via inhalation of dust and fume and via ingestion through contact with lead-contaminated hands, food, cigarettes, and clothing. Absorbed lead accumulates in the body in the soft tissues and bones. Lead is stored in bones for decades, and may cause health effects long after exposure as it is slowly released in the body.

Symptoms of chronic lead poisoning may include headache, joint and muscle aches, weakness, fatigue, irritability, depression, constipation, anorexia, and abdominal discomfort [Moline and Landrigan 2005]. Overexposure to lead has been associated with kidney damage, anemia, high blood pressure, infertility and reduced sex drive in both sexes, and impotence. In most cases, an individual's BLL is a good indication of recent exposure to lead, with a half-life (the time interval it takes for the quantity in the body to be reduced by half its initial value) of 1–2 months [Lauwerys and Hoet 2001; Moline and Landrigan 2005; NCEH 2005]. Elevated zinc protoporphyrin levels have also been used as an indicator of chronic lead intoxication; however, other factors, such as iron deficiency, can cause an elevated zinc protoporphyrin level, so the BLL is a more specific test for evaluating occupational lead exposure.

Under the OSHA general industry lead standard (29 CFR 1910.1025), the PEL for airborne exposure to lead is 50 $\mu g/m^3$ for an 8-hour TWA. The standard requires lowering the PEL for shifts exceeding 8 hours, medical monitoring for employees exposed to airborne lead at or above the action level of 30 $\mu g/m^3$ (8-hour TWA), medical removal of employees whose average BLL is 50 $\mu g/dL$ or greater, and economic protection for medically removed employees. Medically removed employees cannot return to jobs involving lead exposure until their BLL is below 40 $\mu g/dL$. NIOSH has an REL for lead of 50 $\mu g/m^3$ averaged over an 8-hour work shift [NIOSH 2010b]. ACGIH has a TLV for lead of 50 $\mu g/m^3$ (8-hour TWA), with worker BLLs to be controlled to or below 30 $\mu g/dL$, and designation of lead as an animal carcinogen [ACGIH 2012].

The NIOSH REL is consistent with the OSHA PEL, which is intended to maintain worker BLLs below 40 $\mu g/dL$. This is also intended to prevent overt symptoms of lead poisoning, but is not sufficient to protect employees from more subtle adverse health effects like hypertension, renal dysfunction, and reproductive and cognitive effects [Schwartz and Stewart 2007; Schwartz and Hu 2007; Brown-Williams et al. 2009]. Adverse effects on the adult reproductive, cardiovascular, and hematologic systems, and on the development of children of exposed employees, can occur at BLLs as low as 10 $\mu g/dL$ [Sussell 1998]. The Council of State and Territorial Epidemiologists has recommended lowering the definition of elevated blood lead in adults to 10 $\mu g/dL$ to avoid long-term health risks [CSTE 2009].

In homes with a family member occupationally exposed to lead, care must be taken to prevent "take home" of lead, that is, lead carried into the home on clothing, skin, hair, and in vehicles. High BLLs in resident children and elevated concentrations of lead in the house dust have been found in the homes of employees employed in industries associated with high lead exposure [Grandjean and Bach 1986]. Particular effort should be made to ensure that children of persons who work in areas of high lead exposure receive a BLL test. Cognitive and neurological impairment in children from lead exposure is irreversible and can result in lowered intelligence, learning impairment, and behavior issues. CDC has just lowered the reference value for children from 10 to 5 $\mu g/dL$ with evidence showing impairment at even lower levels [MMWR 2012].

Lead-contaminated surface dust represents a potential source of lead exposure, particularly for young children. This may occur either by direct hand-to-mouth contact, or indirectly from hand-to-mouth contact with contaminated clothing, cigarettes, or food. Previous studies have found a significant correlation between resident children's BLLs and house dust lead levels [Farfel and Chisholm 1990]. In the workplace, generally there is little or no correlation between surface lead levels and employee exposures because ingestion exposures are highly dependent on personal hygiene practices and available facilities for maintaining personal hygiene. No current federal standard provides a permissible limit for lead contamination of surfaces in occupational settings.

Ethyl 2-cyanoacrylate

Ethyl 2-cyanoacrylate, which has an unpleasant, acrid odor, is a common ingredient in adhesive super glues. Neither OSHA nor NIOSH has issued OELs for ethyl 2-cyanoacrylate.

The ACGIH TLV (0.2 ppm) is based upon the potential for eye, skin, and upper respiratory tract irritation, dermatitis, and possible respiratory sensitization or asthma [ACGIH 2001]. Although the TLV does not have a skin notation, skin contact has been shown to cause adhesions resulting in tissue damage [ACGIH 2001].

Drugs of Abuse

Methamphetamine, cocaine, heroin, and tetrahydrocannabinol (drugs we sampled for in this evaluation) can produce neurological and physiological effects at relatively high doses (milligram levels) [Gable 2004; DEA 2011]. However, the effects from low doses (nanogram levels of indirect exposure) are not well understood.

Methamphetamine and Cocaine

Methamphetamine and cocaine are classified as stimulants. The possible health effects from an effective dose of stimulants include increased alertness, excitation, euphoria, increased pulse rate and blood pressure, extended wakefulness, and loss of appetite [DEA 2011]. Studies investigating health effects from lower exposures to these compounds are few. In one notable study, investigators administered surveys to law enforcement personnel to determine symptoms experienced while they investigated clandestine methamphetamine laboratories (after ventilation of the laboratories). More than 70% of the respondents reported headaches, central nervous system symptoms, respiratory symptoms, sore throat, and other symptoms. There was also a positive relationship between the number of laboratories investigated and risk of symptoms [Burgess et al. 1996].

Because of the large number of clandestine methamphetamine laboratories requiring remediation, several states have adopted feasibility-based surface contamination limits for methamphetamine. Presently, 16 states have adopted surface contamination limits for methamphetamine ranging from ≤ 100 ng/100 cm^2 to 500 ng/100 cm^2 [NAMSDL 2008]. These limits are intended to prevent adverse health effects to future inhabitants of buildings that once contained clandestine laboratories. Unlike OELs, these limits consider possible exposures to children, who are more susceptible to the health effects of drugs than adults, as well as economic factors associated with remediation. It is reasonable to assume, then, that maintaining surface contamination levels of methamphetamine below these limits should protect the drug evidence laboratory employees from experiencing adverse health effects.

Tetrahydrocannabinol

Tetrahydrocannabinol is the effective drug in marijuana and is classified as cannabis. It is typically smoked. The effects from an effective dose of cannabis can include euphoria, relaxed inhibitions, and disorientation. Short-term health effects may include increased heart rate, coughing from lung irritation, increased appetite, and decreased blood pressure. Long-term users may experience serious health problems such as bronchitis, emphysema, and bronchial asthma. [DEA 2011].

Heroin

Heroin is a rapidly acting opiate often seen as a white or brown powder or as a black sticky substance known as black tar heroin. Heroin can be injected, smoked, or sniffed/snorted. Users report a rush or surge of euphoria, followed by a twilight state of sleep and wakefulness. Health effects can include drowsiness, respiratory depression, nausea, a warm flushing of the skin, dry mouth, and heavy extremities [DEA 2011].

References

ACGIH [2007]. Documentation of the threshold limit values and biological exposure indices. 7th ed. Vol. I. Cincinnati, OH: American Conference of Governmental Industrial Hygienists.

ACGIH [2012]. 2012 TLVs® and BEIs®: threshold limit values for chemical substances and physical agents and biological exposure indices. Cincinnati, OH: American Conference of Governmental Industrial Hygienists.

AIHA [2012]. AIHA 2012 Emergency response planning guidelines (ERPG) & workplace environmental exposure levels (WEEL) handbook. Fairfax, VA: American Industrial Hygiene Association.

Baan R, Grosse Y, Straif K, Secretan B, El Ghissassi F, Bouvard V, Benbrahim-Tallaa L, Guha N, Freeman C, Galichet L, Cogliano V, on the behalf of the WHO International Agency for Research on Cancer Monograph Working Group [2009]. A review of human carcinogens-Part F: chemical agents and related occupations. Lancet Oncol 10(12):1143–1144.

Brown-Williams H, Lichterman J, Kosnett M [2009]. Indecent exposure: lead puts workers and families at risk. Health Research in Action, University of California, Berkeley. Perspectives 4(1)1–9.

Burgess JL, Barnhart S, Checkoway H [1996]. Investigating clandestine drug laboratories: adverse medical effects in law enforcement personnel. Am J Ind Med 30(4):488–494.

CDC [2012]. Guidelines for safe work practices in human and animal medical diagnostic laboratories. MMWR 61(1):38–46.

Chan P, Ho K, Kan K, Stuhmiller J [2001]. Evaluation of impulse noise criteria using human volunteer data. J Acoust Soc America 110(4):1967–1975.

CFR. Code of Federal Regulations. Washington, DC: U.S. Government Printing Office, Office of the Federal Register.

CSTE [2009]. Public health reporting and national notification for elevated blood lead levels. CSTE position statement 09-OH-02. Atlanta, GA: Council of State and Territorial Epidemiologists [http://c.ymcdn.com/sites/www.cste.org/resource/resmgr/PS/09-OH-02.pdf]. Date accessed: February 2013.

DEA [2011]. Drugs of abuse, 2011 edition: a DEA resource guide. [http://www.justice.gov/dea/docs/drugs_of_abuse_2011.pdf]. Date accessed: February 2013.

DHHS [2011]. Addendum to the 12th report on carcinogens. U.S. Department of Health and Human Services, National Toxicology Program. [http://ntp.niehs.nih.gov/ntp/roc/twelfth/Addendum.pdf]. Date accessed: February 2013.

Farfel MR, Chisholm JJ [1990]. Health and environmental outcomes of traditional and modified practices for abatement of residential lead–based paint. Am J Pub Health *80*(10):1240–1245.

Gable RS [2004]. Comparison of acute lethal toxicity of commonly abused psychoactive substances. Addiction *99*(6):686–696.

Grandjean P, Bach E [1986]. Indirect exposures: the significance of bystanders at work and at home. Am Ind Hyg Assoc J *47*(12):819–824.

Green F, Yoshida K [1990]. Characteristics of aerosols generated during autopsy procedures and their potential role as carriers of infectious agents. Occup Environ Hyg *5*(12):853–858.

Gressel MG, Hughes RT [1992]. Effective local exhaust ventilation for controlling formaldehyde exposures during embalming. Appl Occup Environ Hyg *7*(12):840–845.

Howard J [2008]. Prevention through design–introduction. J Saf Res *39*(2):113.

Le SD, Taylor RW, Vidal D, Lovas JJ, Ting E [1992]. Occupational exposure to cocaine involving crime lab personnel. J Forensic Sci *37*(4):959–968.

Lauwerys RR, Hoet P [2001]. Industrial chemical exposure: guidelines for biological monitoring. 3rd ed. Boca Raton, FL: CRC Press, LLC, pp. 21–180.

Lemen RA [1987]. Official letter from RA Lemen, Director, Division of Standards Development and Technology Transfer, National Institute for Occupational Safety and Health, U.S. Department of Health and Human Services, Cincinnati, OH to Tom Hall, Docket Office, Department of Labor, Washington, DC, February 9.

MMWR [2012]. Announcement: response to the Advisory Committee on Childhood Lead Poisoning Prevention Report, low level lead exposure harms children: a renewed call for primary prevention. Atlanta, GA: U.S. Department of Health and Human Services, CDC. [http://www.cdc.gov/mmwr/preview/mmwrhtml/mm6120a6.htm?s_cid=mm6120a6_e%0d%0a]. Date accessed: February 2013.

Moline JM, Landrigan PJ [2005]. Lead. In: Rosenstock L, Cullen MR, Brodkin CA, Redlich CA, eds. Textbook of clinical occupational and environmental medicine. 2nd ed. Philadelphia, PA: Elsevier Saunders, pp. 967–979.

NAMSDL [2008]. State feasibility-based standards. Alexandria, VA: National Alliance for Model State Drug Laws (NAMSDL) [http://www.namsdl.org/documents/RemediationStandardChartFinal.pdf]. Date accessed: February 2013.

NCEH [2005]. Third national report on human exposure to environmental chemicals. Atlanta, GA: U.S. Department of Health and Human Services, Centers for Disease Control and Prevention. National Center for Environmental Health Publication No. 05–0570.

NIOSH [1981]. Current intelligence bulletin 34 – formaldehyde: evidence of carcinogenicity. Cincinnati, OH: U.S. Department of Health and Human Services, Centers for Disease Control, National Institute for Occupational Safety and Health. DHHS (NIOSH) Publication No. DHHS (NIOSH) 81-111 (1981, updated 1997).

NIOSH [1995]. NIOSH recommended exposure limit policy. September 1995. In: NIOSH policy statements. Cincinnati, OH: U.S. Department of Health and Human Services, Centers for Disease Control and Prevention, National Institute for Occupational Safety and Health.

NIOSH [1997]. Health hazard evaluation report: Los Angeles County Department of Coroner – Los Angeles, California. By Martinez K and Tubbs R. Cincinnati, OH: U.S. Department of Health and Human Services, Centers for Disease Control and Prevention, National Institute for Occupational Safety and Health, NIOSH HETA No. 1996-0019-2666.

NIOSH [1998a]. NIOSH hazard control: controlling formaldehyde exposures during embalming. By Gressel M, Votaw A, Hagedorn RT, Flesch JP. Cincinnati, OH: U.S. Department of Health and Human Services, Centers for Disease Control and Prevention, National Institute for Occupational Safety and Health, DHHS (NIOSH) Publication No. 1998-149.

NIOSH [1998b]. Criteria for a recommended standard: occupational noise exposure (revised criteria 1998). Cincinnati, OH: U.S. Department of Health and Human Services, Centers for Disease Control and Prevention, National Institute for Occupational Safety and Health, DHHS (NIOSH) Publication No. 98-126.

NIOSH [2001]. Work related hearing loss. Cincinnati, OH: U.S. Department of Health and Human Services, Centers for Disease Control and Prevention, National Institute for Occupational Safety and Health, DHHS (NIOSH) Publication No. 2001-103.

NIOSH [2009]. NIOSH alert: preventing occupational exposures to lead and noise at indoor firing ranges. By Kardous C, King B, Khan A, Whelan E, Tubbs R, Barsan M, Crouch K, Murphy W, Willson R, Esswein E, Boeniger M. Cincinnati, OH: U.S. Department of Health and Human Services, Centers for Disease Control and Prevention, National Institute for Occupational Safety and Health, DHHS (NIOSH) Publication No. 2009-136.

NIOSH [2010a]. NIOSH manual of analytical methods, 4th ed. Schlecht PC, O'Connor PF, eds. Cincinnati, OH: U.S. Department of Health and Human Services, Centers for Disease Control and Prevention, National Institute for Occupational Safety and Health, DHHS (NIOSH) Publication 94–113 August 1994); 1st Supplement Publication 96–135, 2nd Supplement Publication 98–119; 3rd Supplement 2003–154. [http://www.cdc.gov/niosh/nmam/]. Date accessed: February 2013.

NIOSH [2010b]. NIOSH pocket guide to chemical hazards. Cincinnati, OH: U.S. Department of Health and Human Services, Centers for Disease Control and Prevention, National Institute for Occupational Safety and Health, DHHS (NIOSH) Publication No. 2010-168c. [http://www.cdc.gov/niosh/npg/]. Date accessed: February 2013.

NIOSH [2011]. Health hazard evaluation report: evaluation of police officers' exposures to chemicals while working inside a drug vault – Kentucky. By Fent KW, Durgam S, West C, Gibbins J, Smith J. Cincinnati, OH: U.S. Department of Health and Human Services, Centers for Disease Control and Prevention, National Institute for Occupational Safety and Health, NIOSH HETA No. 2010-0017-3133.

Nolte K, Taylor D, Richmond J [2002]. Biosafety consideration for autopsy. Am J Forensic Med Pathol 23(2):107–122.

NRC [1981]. Formaldehyde and other aldehydes. National Research Council (National Academy Press), Washington, DC.

OSHA [1985]. OSHA method 55: methyl-2-cyanoacrylate and ethyl-2-cyanoacrylate. In: Sampling and analytical methods. Salt Lake City, Utah: U.S. Department of Labor, Occupational Safety and Health Administration, Organic Methods Evaluation Branch. [www.osha.gov/dts/sltc/methods/index.html]. Date accessed: February 2013.

Perry J, Parker G, Jagger J [2003]. Scalpel blades: reducing injury risk. Adv Exposure Prev 6(4):37–40.

Schwartz BS, Hu H [2007]. Adult lead exposure: time for change. Environ Health Perspect 115(3):451–454.

Schwartz BS, Stewart WF [2007]. Lead and cognitive function in adults: a question and answers approach to a review of the evidence for cause, treatment, and prevention. Int Rev Psychiatry 19(6):671–692.

Smith J, Sammons D, Robertson S, Biagini R, Snawder J [2010]. Measurement of multiple drugs in urine, water, and on surfaces using fluorescence covalent microbead immunosorbent assay. Toxicol Mech Methods 20(9):587–593.

Sussell A [1998]. Protecting workers exposed to lead-based paint hazards: a report to Congress. Cincinnati, OH: U.S. Department of Health and Human Services, Centers for Disease Control and Prevention, National Institute for Occupational Safety and Health, DHHS (NIOSH) Publication No. 98–112.

Keywords: NAICS 922120 (Police Protection) and 923120 (Administration of Public Health Programs), coroner, autopsies, histology, firearms, fingerprints, drugs, evidence, formaldehyde, lead, ethyl 2-cyanoacrylate, cocaine, marijuana, methamphetamine, heroin, surface contamination

The Health Hazard Evaluation Program investigates possible health hazards in the workplace under the authority of Section 20(a)(6) of the Occupational Safety and Health Act of 1970, 29 U.S.C. 669(a)(6). The Health Hazard Evaluation Program also provides, upon request, technical assistance to federal, state, and local agencies to control occupational health hazards and to prevent occupational illness and disease. Regulations guiding the Program can be found in Title 42, Code of Federal Regulations, Part 85; Requests for Health Hazard Evaluations (42 CFR 85).

Acknowledgments

Analytical Support: Jennifer Roberts, Jerry Smith, Deborah Sammons, John Snawder, and Bureau Veritas North America (Fort Lauderdale, Florida)
Desktop Publishers: Greg Hartle and Mary Winfree
Editor: Ellen Galloway
Health Communicator: Stefanie Brown
Industrial Hygiene Field Assistance: Steven Ahrenholz
Logistics: Donnie Booher and Karl Feldmann

Availability of Report

Copies of this report have been sent to the employer, employees, and union at the facility. The state and local health department and the Occupational Safety and Health Administration Regional Office have also received a copy. This report is not copyrighted and may be freely reproduced.

This report is available at http://www.cdc.gov/niosh/hhe/reports/pdfs/2011-0146-3170.pdf.

Recommended citation for this report:
NIOSH [2013]. Health hazard evaluation report: evaluation of potential employee exposures during crime and death investigations at a county coroner's office. By King B, Musolin K, Choi J. Cincinnati, OH: U.S. Department of Health and Human Services, Centers for Disease Control and Prevention, National Institute for Occupational Safety and Health, NIOSH HETA No. 2011-0146-3170.